MODITA VAN ZUMMEREN

DEPRESSION

A STEPPING-STONE TOWARDS BLISS

Beyond Depression with Consciousness

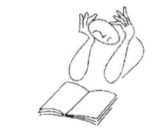

Aspekt Publishers

Depression a Stepping-stone towards Bliss
Original Title: *Depressie, een Opstap naar Geluk*
© Modita van Zummeren
© 2018 Uitgeverij Aspekt
Amersfoortsestraat 27, 3769 AD Soesterberg, The Nederlands
info@uitgeverijaspekt.nl www.uitgeverijaspekt.nl

Translation: Modita van Zummeren & Bodhigita Jane Marshall
Cover Design: Mark Heuveling, Snezhina Uzunova
Editing and Production: Mark Heuveling

Texts from Osho with permission from Osho International Foundation, www.osho.com/copyrights.
OSHO® is a registered Trademark of Osho International Foundation, www.osho.com/trademarks

ISBN: 9789463385152
NUR: 130

No part of this publication may be reproduced, stored in a retrieval system, or transmitted in any form or by any means, electronic, mechanical, photocopying, recording, or otherwise, without written permission of the publisher.

DEPRESSION *A STEPPING-STONE TOWARDS BLISS*

I dedicate this book to

my beloved source of inspiration Meera Hashimoto

&

to my beloved master Osho

Contents

	Poem: the steppe will flower	11
	Introduction	13
1	Accepting Depression	17

Part 1: My Experience of Depression — **23**

2	How my depression developed	25
3	My final depression begins	67
4	A day in my depression	69
5	The turning point in my depression	77
6	A day in my happy life	97

Part 2: Taking the Helm into your Own Hands — **103**

7	The value of taking responsibility for yourself	105
8	The illusion of antidepressants	113
9	Saying 'yes' is opening yourself to life	125
10	Stopping comparing yourself with others brings you back to yourself	135

Part 3: Healing from the Body   **143**

11   Your body is the basis of good therapy   145

12   Physical exercise with awareness   161

13   Food and Depression   167

Part 4: Family Constellations   **181**

14   Family Constellations   183
      Becoming the child of your parents again

Part 5: The importance of Osho Meditations   **193**

15   OSHO® Active Meditations   195

16   OSHO® Meditative Therapies   209

Part 6: Re-establishment of the Connection with Yourself and the Other   **231**

17   Being connected and in contact with the other   233

Part 7: Passion and Connection with the Soul   **251**

18   Passion and Meaning   253

19   Listening to your Soul   265

Last word	273
About the author	277
Word of thanks	279
Selected Bibliography	285

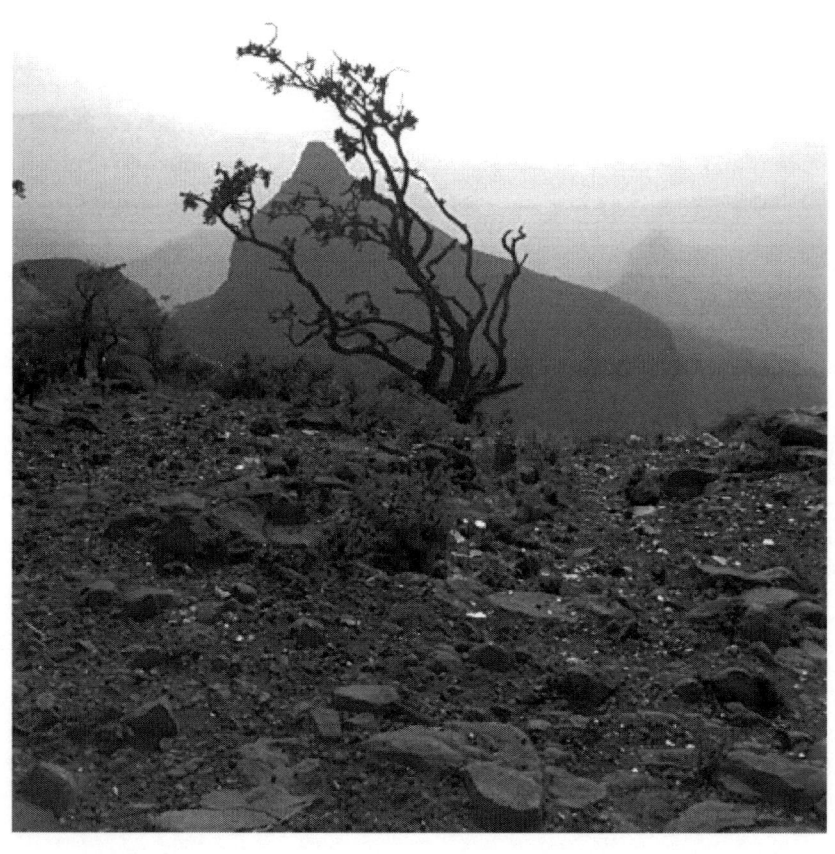

*The dead man will live.
The dead man will hear: live now.
Gone to the very end and buried under stones:
dead man, dead man, get up,
the light of the morning.*

*A hand will beckon us,
a voice will call us: "I open
heaven and earth and abyss"
and we will hear
and they will get up
and laugh and cheer and live.*

*Huub Oosterhuis**

---

* Translated from www.gedichtensite.nl

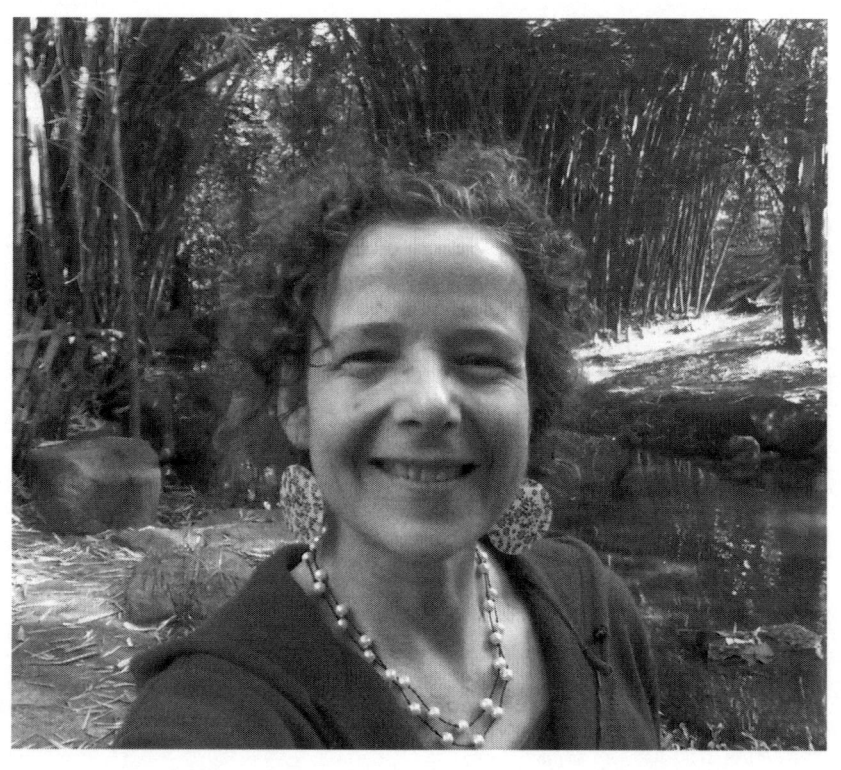

INTRODUCTION

This book contains some keys to come out of depression with consciousness and without medicines.

These keys I didn't learn in my medical education. As a doctor of medicine you are trained in the DSM handbook, in which psychic disorders are categorised by a couple of prescribed criteria. You learn which antidepressant to prescribe for which clinical picture, not knowing that - except in severe depressions - these medicines don't work at all and that they are mainly put on the market by the pharmaceutical industry to make a lot of money. Medical doctors are not educated in the importance of healthy food, the influence of the heart on the balance of the nervous system or the message of the soul in psychic diseases. Nor is the influence of the family system taken into consideration.

The working method in conventional medicine is still too much focused on the fight against symptoms and not enough on the re-establishment of a healthy balance of body and mind.

My depressions put me on to a search for a way to heal myself through consciousness and this search brought me via gestalt-therapy and Zen meditation to India, where I became inspired by the Indian mystic Osho. He brought me into contact with my *being* and from there into connection with the whole life of which I am part.

He has given me insight to myself and his Active Meditations have made it possible for me to transform my negativity into a 'yes' to life.

As well as this, I discovered through Family Constellations in Art Therapy Training with Meera Hashimoto that my depression was rooted in unsolved issues belonging to my family system.

This book is addressed to everyone who is depressed and who wants to go beyond depression by raising his or her consciousness. If one is ready to face and to struggle through the dark parts inside him/herself, then depression can become a stepping-stone towards bliss.

This book is also for family members, friends, doctors and therapists close to the person who is depressed; to widen the point of view around depression and to enhance understanding for the passage through which a depressed person is going; a passage which is not easy, but which, when it has been struggled through, gives a bliss that is bigger than has ever been known before.

The keys which I give in this book are keys to unlock the heart, the soul and the *being*. The approaches from the different chapters reinforce each other.

The causes of the depression have mostly developed over many, many years. Patience, love and compassion are needed to investigate, pass through and finally transform the depression.

This can only happen from an attitude of acceptance of the depression. That's what the first chapter is about.

I dedicate this book to my master, the Indian mystic Osho, who has shown me the way to follow myself and the way to an attitude of a full 'yes' towards both life and death. In his presence I feel the highest potential of the human being: celebrating existence from moment to moment, resting in oneself and being connected with the whole universe.

I also dedicate this book to Meera Hashimoto, Japanese artist and artist of life, who developed Osho Art Therapy, through which she has connected many people throughout the world with their creativity, with meditation and with their own life-energy. In February 2017 she left her body. Her work is continued by her students.

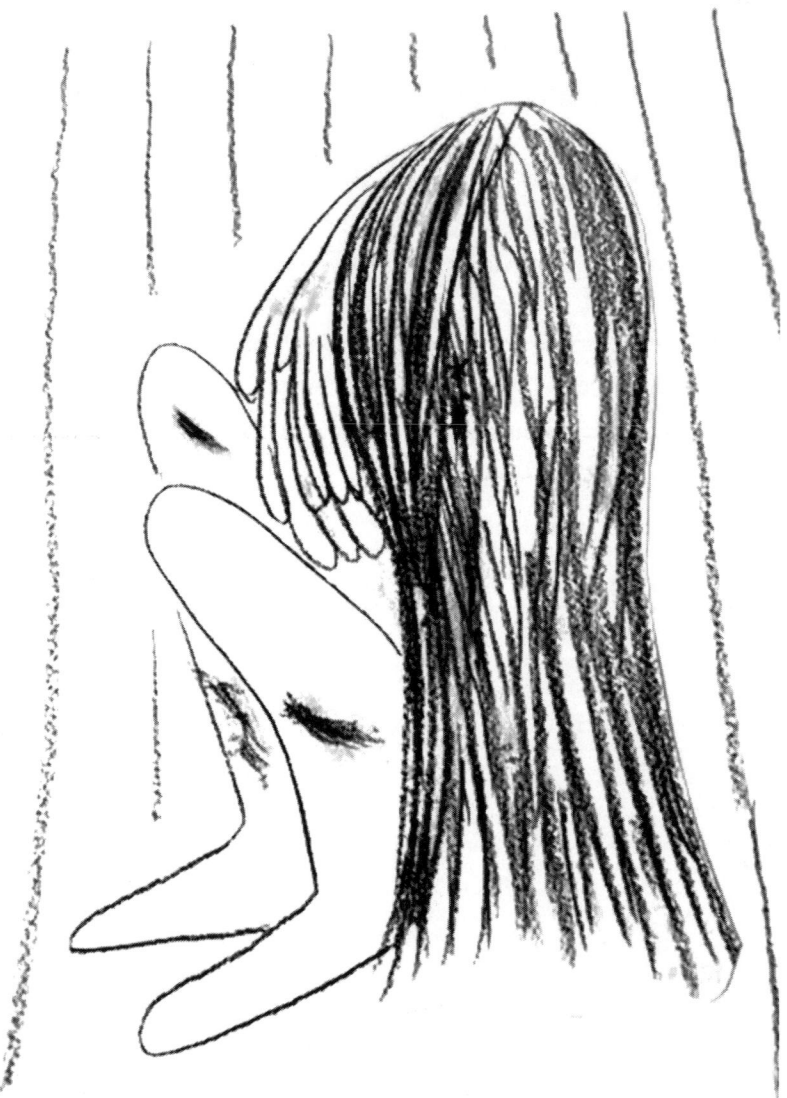

1 ACCEPTING DEPRESSION

Many depressive people remain stuck in their depression because they try to avoid reaching the deepest point of the ditch. Unfortunately there is no way to really be cured without going through the deepest part of the valley. *

Willem van de Sanden

The first thing I did when a depression arose was: I fought. I did my utmost to prevent this emotional assassin from putting me down this time. Each time I failed in this, my discouragement got bigger.

To overcome depression it is first of all necessary to accept it. For this courage and trust are needed.

---

* Willem van de Sanden, psychologist and psychotherapist - Author of the Dutch book *Depressie actief overwinnen [Active Overcoming Depression]*

If you are depressed, so be depressed

Osho says about this:

"Remember this: whenever you are depressed, wait for the moment that the depression goes. Nothing lasts forever: the depression will go. When the depression leaves you, wait - be aware and alert - because after the depression, after this night, there will be a dawn, the sun will rise. If you can be alert in that moment, you will be happy that you were depressed. You will be grateful that you were depressed because only through that depression, this possibility; only through that depression, this moment of happiness.

But what do we do? - we move in an infinite regression. We get depressed because of the depression: a second depression follows. If you are depressed, that's okay, nothing is wrong in it. It is beautiful because through it you will learn and mature. But then you feel badly: 'Why do I get depressed? I should not get depressed.' Then you start fighting with the depression. The real depression is good, but the second depression is unreal - and this unreal depression will cloud your mind. You will miss the moment that would have followed the real depression.

"When depressed, be depressed. Don't get depressed about your depression. When depressed, simply be depressed. Don't fight it, don't create any diversion; don't force it to go. Just allow it to happen, it will go by itself. Life is a flux, nothing remains. You are not needed: the river moves by itself, you are not to push it. If you are trying to push it, you are simply foolish. The river flows by itself - allow it to flow.

"When there is a depression, allow it to be. Don't get depressed about it. If you want to remove it sooner, you will get depressed. If you fight it, you will create a secondary depression, which is dangerous. The first depression is beautiful, God-given. The second depression is your own. It is not God-given, it is mental. Then you will move in mental grooves - they are infinite.

"If you get depressed, be happy that you are depressed and allow the depression to be. Then, suddenly the depression will disappear and there will be a breakthrough. There will be no clouds and the sky will be clear. For a single moment, heaven opens for you. If you are not depressed about your depression you can contact, you can commune, you can enter this heavenly gate. And once you know it, you have learned one of the ultimate laws of life: life uses the opposite as a teacher, as a background."*

If you are depressed, allow the depression to be

Pamela Kribbe is a Dutch graduate philosopher and also a medium. In her book *Nacht van de Ziel [Night of the Soul]* she describes how the way to make your soul shine in your life is to go first towards the darkness in yourself, which longs to be resolved:

"In the depression we meet our dark sides in a very confrontational way. What we have to do is to face this darkness in the first instance. Only then can it resolve and you can experience your light in all its fullness.

"If it is difficult for you to accept and bless negative energies that torment you, then let them appear to you as a child that is searching for help. If you struggle with fear, if you ask

---

* Osho - *The New Alchemy: To Turn You On #8*

yourself if life on this earth is meaningful at all, let those voices take the form of a desperate child. See the heaviest emotion before you as the face of a child, which exactly expresses what you are feeling. Then feel your own strength and stretch out your hand to the child. Bless it. Feel who *you* are. You are the parent and guide of the child. That is the true relation between you and your heaviest emotions. The night of your soul invites you to take the hand of the child in you, who carries the heaviest emotions. It needs your help. Accompany it, console it and encourage it, but don't forget who you are. You are the loving parent, the wise guide, who sees farther than the child, across the threshold." *

The Night of your Soul invites you to take the child in you, who carries the heaviest emotions, by the hand

---

Depression is often a Mourning Process

Darian Leader, British psychoanalyst, sees with his patients that much of what we call depression nowadays is in fact mourning; the reaction to a loss. Loss of a beloved for example or a job or the place where you used to live. In his book *The New Black* he pleads in favour of dropping the whole idea of depression and of looking at how we can deal with our losses. Often we want to overcome them, but when something that we loved has been lost, it will always remain a part of us. It is then rather a question of integrating the loss into our life.

---

* Pamela Kribbe - *Dark Night of the Soul*

Depressed = Deep rest

Jeff Foster, who experienced depression himself, gives a beautiful interview on YouTube about depression:

"We can view depression not as a mental illness, but on a deeper level as a profound and very misunderstood state of deep rest, which we enter when we are completely exhausted by the weight of our own false story of ourselves.

"There is a truth to depression and this truth we often miss in our urge to quickly cure depression; you are sad and quickly you make yourself happy or get back to work.

"Actually we can so quickly end up missing the deeper truth of depression, which is: this isn't your life to hold up; this story of me and my life. This isn't who you really are. This person, that you are pretending to be, this character that you are pretending to be, this facade that you are living in the world, it's not really who you are. You have been pretending to be something that you are not.

"So this is going to crush you. Pretending to be something that you are not. Pretending to be this image. Pretending to be the-story-of-me is eventually going to become exhausting for everyone. And in the case of clinical depression it can even become totally exhausting and crushing. But the point is that it is not about holding up your life in the first place. This story is not who you are. It's not who you really are. So that's the deeper truth of depression.

"So perhaps depression is not a sickness or an illness. Perhaps it's an invitation. I often say: life is a constant invitation to awaken or an invitation to discover who you really are."*

---

* Jeff Foster, Youtube: *From 'De-pressed' to 'Deep Rest'*

Depression is an invitation
to discover who you really are

In the next five chapters I will describe my personal experience of depression.

Part 1

My Experience of Depression

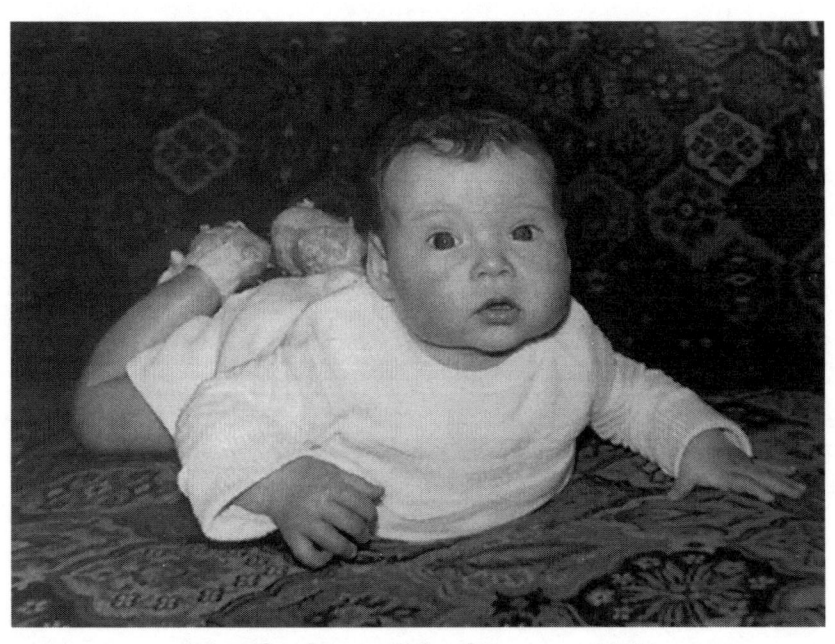

Marijke, born 24th of January 1962

2 HOW MY DEPRESSION DEVELOPED

"Many people, highly sensitive persons for sure, ask themselves what their vocation is. Next they start thinking about what it could be. But in that thinking lurks a big pitfall. Namely, your vocation is found in a deeper layer of yourself: your soul. And that will not easily be addressed by thinking. Your soul will be especially addressed by intuition, by feeling. So you have to discover intuitively what your vocation is."*

Anonymous

The story of my depression starts even before I am born. I lose my twin sister in the womb. My mother tells me only once when I am a child that when she is pregnant with me, the family doctor hears two little hearts beating. She tells how she immediately starts knitting: two small sweaters, four small socks. And then, weeks afterwards, only one heart can be heard: mine. My twin sister has died. It is the loss of the one with whom I have had the most tender connection before my birth.

---

* Anonymous, www.hooggevoelig.nl

I come into the world with a feeling of guilt: I am alive, but my twin sister is not. Until my final depression I keep searching for her from deep inside me and I want to be where my twin sister is. And that is not on this earth.

---
*I want to be where my twin sister is
and that is not on this earth*

I am born from a strong woman, who carries a lot of pain. She is born in Indonesia, where she grows up in an abundant Nature with gaudy green rice fields and high mountains. She is always outside; her house doesn't even have windows and with dexterous hands she plays at knucklebones with her friends, brothers and sisters.

Then a drastic change happens: the war breaks out - the Japanese have invaded. The whole family is allowed to take with them only one small suitcase before they enter the overloaded train, heading for the concentration camp. The family cannot stay together; her father has to go to Burma, to work there under the watchful eye of the Japanese on the railways, from where almost nobody returns alive. Many of his comrades die there. He himself survives. He manages not to die from exhaustion during the devastating long marches by taking care to start the walk at the front and to finish at the end of the line. When the war is over, he is not on the list of survivors that reaches my mother's camp. But later, neither does he appear to be on the list of the dead men.

Then, a man who comes back from Burma visits the camp of my mother and her sisters, and tells them about a man with a long beard who can stand on one hand. They immediately know that this is their father and they go by boat to Bangkok to pick him up.

However, at the beginning of the war, the rest of the family is transported by armoured train to one of the concentration camps. My mother's eldest brother has to go to the boys' camp, because he is more than ten years old. Her mother, youngest brother and four sisters all stay together. Her mother remains most of the time in the sick-bay of the camp due to severe intestinal infections. One day, when she is close to death, she is saved by a syringe with medicines somehow obtained by her doctor.

Every day the dead bodies of the children, with whom my mother was playing just a short time before - and who have died because of malnutrition - are loaded on a wooden cart and driven out of the camp. My mother describes how sad it is for her when a baby, which she used to love very much, dies and is carried away in a shoe box.

Almost everybody has worm infections. My mother hates it when the long eel-worms pass out of her anus.

In the camp they live in one house with other families. My mother's family lives in the kitchen and my mother sleeps in a small kitchen-cupboard, because of lack of space.

In the morning she is given a tasteless paste. The rest of the day some rice; less than fills the centre of the palm of the hand. She is always hungry. If I say as a child that I am hungry, my mother says that I don't know what that means. Even today I hardly dare to say that I am hungry. In this way I lose the trust in the signals that my body gives me.

I have lost the trust in the signals that my body gives

My mother's youngest sister always has a small cushion bound around her buttocks, because her sitting bones are almost sticking through her skin and this allows her still to be able to sit.

Sometimes my mother finds a frog, which she eats alive. If the Japanese were to see this she would be caned, so if they approach she quickly digs a little hole in the ground with her foot, drops the frog in, then closes the hole with her foot quick as lightning. High barbed wire surrounds the camp. When the children do something wrong, their mother is punished by the Japanese: she has to sit then in the burning sun for hours with a stick clamped between the hollows of the knees. Many mothers die because of this or are terribly burnt by the sun. So the children are always on their guard.

Every day there is the parade: for hours they are lined up in rows, so that the Japanese can see if everybody is present. When the Japanese pass by, they have to bow down, which they experience as very humiliating. In the daytime they work hard in the fields. The girls are in danger of being raped by the Japanese. For her whole life my mother is afraid of bodily contact.

The whole family survives the war. My mother's eldest brother joins his mother and sisters again. Together they go by boat to Thailand to pick up their father. When they have found him they sail on to the Netherlands, where their parents come from originally.

They are not received there with a warm welcome. The Second World War is just over and everybody thinks that the colonists simply had a wonderful time over there in Indonesia. They could not get support from anyone for their traumas. They store everything that has happened somewhere deep in their brain and lock it away as firmly as possible. Later, when I work in an asylum-seeker-centre as a medical doctor, a psychiatrist there says that this is the best thing they could have done: to screw the lid of the cesspool down as strongly as they could and then build up a life - a house, a family, work - so that they had a foundation on which they could bear living.

My mother survives by not feeling anything

When my mother arrives in the Netherlands she is fifteen years old. Everything she has experienced separates her from her peers as they hit puberty and she has no common point to connect her with them. So she keeps quiet.

In 2013 I go with my sisters to the documentary *Buitenkampers Boekan Main* by Hetty Naaijkens- Retel Helmrich. It tells the story of the Dutch Indonesians who lived outside the camps during the Japanese occupation. Hetty, a second generation war victim like me, describes how the first generation war victims suppress all emotion in order to survive, and do not feel. The second generation (to which I belong) carries all these emotions and is tasked with having to process them at some point.

Because their house in the Netherlands has yet to be built, my mother and her sisters are sent to a boarding school run by nuns. Her father sets off to Indonesia again for four years in order to qualify for his pension.

The boarding school is even worse for my mother than the concentration camp. The nuns see to it that my mother and her sisters are separated from each other. She has to shower under a plastic cape to hide her body, letters from her mother are intercepted and she and her sisters are called thieves, because the nuns have heard that they have stolen food from the Japanese in the camp. (My mother had scraped, together with her eldest sister, food scraps from the cooking pots of the Japanese - which were put outside the kitchen - to share with the rest of the family).

My mother has missed the whole of High School in the camp. Her dream is to become a primary school teacher and she starts teacher training school. With tremendous perseverance she continues studying at night. Because the nuns have forbidden study in the evening, she has to do it secretly with a torch under her blanket.

Her dream to become a primary school teacher gives her strength

---

Her second dream is to have a family and children. She puts a contact advertisement in the school magazine and in this way meets my father, who is also working as a teacher. She is deliriously happy when first I and later also my three sisters are born. They call me Marijke, which soon becomes Marij. Later, in the Osho Meditation Centre I receive the name Modita.

I grow up in Bergeijk, a small village near the Belgian border, and live in a double world: a visible and an invisible one. The visible world is the fairytale world my mother creates, with beautiful stories and fairy tales which she tells me before going to sleep: goblin houses which we build in the sandpit with small paths, and on which we find a chocolate bar the next morning, 'from the goblins'. On Saint Nicholas morning our dolls are dressed with clothes knitted by my mother, their hair is combed beautifully and the presents are all displayed on one of the chairs of the lounge suite.

The invisible world is underneath. That is woven out of my mother's stories from the camp: stories about hunger and death, the humiliation by the Japanese and the imprisonment behind the barbed wire.

My living environment looks safe but in the background I feel that there is something horrific.

Deep inside I feel that the world is unsafe

When I am nine years old my trust in adults reaches a breaking point. In the Netherlands, children are told that Saint Nicholas comes on a boat from Spain every year in November to leave presents for children on the fifth of December: but my school teacher says that Saint Nicholas doesn't exist. My fairy tale world breaks down. I go home and tell my mother that the teacher has told us the date when Saint Nicholas died. My mother says that Saint Nicholas was such a good person that he could return from Heaven to Earth. From that moment on I am split between my mother and the teacher. I choose my mother. I feel how important it is for her that the fairy tale world remains and until I am twelve I pretend still to believe in Saint Nicholas.

My mother tells me that everyone receives a vocation in his or her life. For her it was that of primary school teacher. From eleven onwards I worry if I will ever hear my vocation. When I walk to school, I listen with my head tilted towards the sky. But it remains silent.

As the end of my primary school period comes closer I become more and more afraid of what will come next. My mother entered the concentration camp when she was eleven years old. Something in me senses that she doesn't know how life should look beyond that age in a situation without war. In my head circles: 'after Primary School my life will be finished'.

I think that my life will be finished after Primary School

It is a mammoth undertaking for me to go to high school. Because my mother considers it very bad that children there don't play anymore, I keep on playing, to support her and to prove that it is possible. I am laughed at. Fiercely I throw myself upon my homework then; that gives me a good excuse to withdraw from social life. Where I had friends in primary school, now very soon I find myself socially isolated.

When I am sixteen years old, my family doctor notices a strange-looking scar on my mother's arm. A previous family doctor had simply burned away a mole there without investigating it further. The new doctor finds it necessary to get the scar - and a big area around it - removed. Investigation of the removed tissue shows that it is indeed a melanoma: cancer of a mole. This diagnosis is not communicated to my mother. She discovers it later by herself when she asks for the report of the analysis.

The melanoma is black and the skin is a contact-organ. I think that her cancer has to do with the fact that the Japanese wore black gloves to avoid infection when they touched the Dutch, and with the fact that she was standing in the burning sun for such a long time during the daily parade in the Japanese concentration camp.

That same year my parents have started renovating our house. The kitchen changes into a desert of sand with shelves to cross it; goodbye, feelings of cosiness. At the same time I am maturing as an adolescent and in the changing room of the gymnasium at the high school someone makes a derogatory remark about my slightly growing belly. I ask my mother, who is slim - and therefore an example for me - how she is able to remain so slender. She hesitates before answering. She says that she never eats many desserts. From that moment on I drop all sweet things and also start economising on other nutrition. I am proud of myself; it's astonishingly quick to lose weight, and proudly I tell my mother a few weeks later that I have already lost four kilos. She looks worried. I continue losing weight without sharing anymore with my mother. My days have a purpose now: avoiding calories and losing weight. Soon I reach a body weight of forty kilos. I don't lose more than this because I feel it could cost my life. I don't have feelings anymore; everything is uniform, grey, and emotionless. It is greyish and safe at the same time; I don't have to feel any longer the pain which has always invisibly been around me. The connection with my mother consists of a daily struggle around food. It is upsetting to feel how much pain she has because of it. I smuggle away that feeling. My hormonal growth stands still. I am happy about that, because I don't want to have an adult female body. My mother has told me once that she did not have menstruation any more in the concentration camp because of underfeeding and that seems to me a positive side effect of eating very little

By eating hardly anything I do not have to feel any more

In drawings, which I leave openly on my study table, I scream for help: I paint myself in a public square with high walls with small watch-windows, stretching out my arms to the people who are free outside those walls and who are running speedily away from me.

One day my mother silently enters my room and gives me a book: 'The Golden Cage'.* I read it and cry in recognition. Now I know that what I have is called 'anorexia' and I also know now that my mother knows.

My father is a very loving, conscientious man. His handicap concerns his eyes; he has almost all the possible eye diseases which you can have and he suffers mainly from the fact that reading is difficult for him. When he is eighteen years old he goes to Brazil to study to be a priest. Because of the rapid worsening of his eyesight he has to return to the Netherlands after three years, where he first becomes a primary school teacher and after that a teacher of mathematics. He comes from a family of 'don't air your dirty laundry in public' and although I feel blessed by his love, I miss him emotionally. In the many fights at the table between my mother and me, my father seems to be absent. From the expression on his face I see how heavily he takes it to heart, but he remains quiet and goes cycling. He minds a lot that everyone can see from my thinness that something is wrong with us at home.

Also my father remains quiet about his emotions

When I get my diploma at the end of the high school, I am not happy. I realise that every top mark I have got has a high

---

* Hilde Bruch - *The Golden Cage*

cost; that of having studied far too much without really living.

I don't know what further education I will enter. Text books sicken me after so much time spent on them, and they do not provide what I long for – something beyond the mere mechanical explanation of the world, which misses the mystery. In this last school year there has been one moment which transcends this mechanical world. It is when my teacher of Biology says, after describing the fusion of the egg with the sperm cell: 'and then there is the mystery'. A silence drops in the class at that, and I feel wonder at the mystery; I wonder about something which is more than what you can see with the naked eye; this is what I want to be connected with. At that moment I want to study biology, but I reflect on the fact that I cannot earn money that way. I choose then to study medicine with the question in my head: 'I wonder how they will make me a medical doctor within eight years'. I see a doctor as a kind of magician, who recognises the diagnosis as soon as his patient enters his consulting room. But deep inside I don't know what I want. I have often since had the feeling that my choice to be a doctor has had to do with something from a past life; with something that I have to do which lies at the foundation of health: first, healing purulent wounds. Does it have to do with the concentration camp in which my mother was? Does it have to do with what I learn later: that my mother had wanted to become a doctor, but was not allowed to do so because there was no money? First I am not selected as a student. The whole summer I sit soullessly on the sofa, not knowing what to do. Because of my high marks I am allowed to draw lots once again for Medicine and I am admitted.

The first day of College I am sitting with three hundred other students in a wooden lecture theatre, where the circular benches reach to the ceiling. It is dark, so that one can see the electrical lights that are moving over a giant model of a heart. In this way one can see how the electric impulses are spread over the organ. I feel very miserable with the mechanical view of the human body. There is no psychology, philosophy or ethics in my curriculum. Because I still hardly eat, I don't have many feelings or emotions. On top of all this an image of the human is added now, reduced to a collection of bones, muscles and chemical structures. Nevertheless I throw myself, just like in high school, into doing nothing apart from studying, and my social isolation carries on in the city of Utrecht.

My social isolation carries on in the city of Utrecht

I don't dare to stop my studies, because I don't know what I would do then, so I continue. In the second and third year I am fascinated by the miracle of the human body that is built so ingeniously, but mostly I am very sombre.

One day my mother sits down next to me at the kitchen table and asks me how I feel. This is the first time she asks me about my feelings; it is a question which does not have to do with food. I feel seen, touched and very close to her. It is scary also. What should I say? How can I explain it? But most of all: what do I actually feel? What is really mine? Stammering, I utter some sentences which I do not remember any more.

Immediately after this one of my sisters gets anorexia. I feel that I have set the wrong example and feel guilty. At the same time I am angry too, because she outstrips me in being thin.

She gets all the attention now. She goes to the hospital and is seen as sick, whereas I used to be called a stubborn donkey.

Out of joint, I start eating blindly. Or more accurately to gorge; I eat everything I come across, without tasting it. In the supermarket I snatch the granola straight from the packet even before I have reached the check-out. In my student room I spread every slice of a whole loaf of bread with a thick layer of butter, dredge it with sugar and get all the slices down one by one. Next is a packet of chocolate cookies. Wherever I go, the first thing I look for is if there is something to eat. And on Sunday, when all the shops are closed, the shop at the petrol station is still available. I try to fill an insatiable hole. For a moment, when just after the binge eating my belly almost bursts from the multitude of food, this seems to be possible. But two hours later the hole is there again and I regret the gorging, which contributes to my quickly fattening body.

One day my father tells me that he and my mother can't help me anymore; that I have to look for help somewhere else, and that it is better if I don't come home for a while at the weekends because my eating problem is too much of a burden for my mother.

My parents can't help me any more

Feeling empty I go to Utrecht and sign myself up at the secretariat of the psychiatry department of the academic hospital. I am afraid that, without help, my weight will increase way above one hundred kilos.

To my consternation there is a waiting period of three months. They become three very long months. At the weekends I do nothing else but study.

The psychiatrist I get is quite a corpulent middle-aged woman. In the first meeting she measures my weight and finds it too low; as a result my emotions are so much on the back burner that she cannot work with me. I have to gain five kilos.

That is difficult for me to hear but at the same time: eating makes sense to me now. After a few weeks I have reached my target weight and my therapy can start.

My psychiatrist asks me: 'what age do you feel you are?' I am twenty-three years old then. I tell her that I am always taken to be younger, but she wants to hear my own response. Her question makes me feel frozen and helpless. I realise that I don't know anything about myself. The image comes to me of all the puzzle pieces of myself which I have boarded out to others returning, dropping back into my body through my head. I start to cry then. For the first time I feel something that is mine. I experience something of who I am or what refers to who I am.

A few pieces of the puzzle of my feeling come back

Once every two weeks I get therapy now. I dislike my body because I have gained so much weight and I feel the fat bobbling around me like a jelly pudding when I move. But my psychiatrist proves to be right concerning the return of feelings at a higher body weight. That means that now I also feel I don't want to be so isolated anymore.

One day I pick up the third year prospectus of my school of medicine, in which there are a couple of pages with the photos of all the students. I go through them all and choose two girls who seem to be nice. Courageously I approach them after college, and from that moment on we spend a lot of time together.

Nevertheless I feel gloomy most of the time. I am not happy with my studies and I am very little in touch with myself. I keep studying a lot because otherwise I am afraid that I will not become a good doctor. During the Christmas holidays of the fifth year of medicine I burn myself out studying ten hours per day for three months. I have more or less decided to study so much that I will go crazy, so then everyone will be able to see that I have to stop my studies. In my paediatric training period I am so depressed that one day, when I am in my parents' house, I don't want to get out of bed any more. My youngest sister comes to my bedroom in the attic to get me up by playing the flute; she wants me so much to live, and I do not know how to do that.

At that time, the inevitable happens to my mother: she discovers a swollen lymph gland in her armpit beside the removed mole on her arm. I know immediately: her cancer has spread. I think I am guilty of causing this metastasis because just two days before I had said to my previous piano teacher: 'I have to get loose of my mother in a drastic way'.

My mother leaps into the medical loop to start the battle with the melanoma.

I want to stop my studies. I know it for sure: this is not for me. But taking things less radically, I simply report sick. Because I feel that I won't get out of bed if I don't have a daily rhythm and a structure, I sign myself up for the psychiatric unit of a hospital in Eindhoven.

I have need for a structure, otherwise I don't get out of my bed anymore

It bothers my mother a lot that I need to go to that unit. It makes her ask herself what she has done wrong as a mother. Nonetheless, she has the strength to drive me in her car to the psychiatric unit when I want to withdraw from admission later on.

Meanwhile she is busy with the fight with the medical world, which has withheld from her the true information about her sickness. Fighting fiercely for honesty, she makes no secret of her low opinion of conventional medicine. She calls it: 'the white circus'. That is difficult for me to hear as a student doctor.

For three months I stay at the psychiatric unit. During the first days, I want to escape. There are many depressed people, who sit in a corner in the big daycare room from which you almost cannot see the other side because so many people are smoking. An hysterical woman continually lies down on the floor as if she's dead in front of the door of the dining-room. We all have to cross her to be able to reach our lunch. On the second evening I have just decided to leave this desolate place when a woman approaches me, telling me she has been in a coma for a long time and that since reviving from it she has got a different personality which she cannot live with. She indicates that she is finding it terrible in this unit and that she wants to leave. I motivate her to stay and realise that if I say this, I have to stay myself too. So I stay.

I think a lot about the meaninglessness of life and about death. I consider that all life is going to end anyhow when the sun no longer exists after thousands of years and I write in a poem: 'What is the meaning of constantly 'having been' in a world which 'has been' later on?' In my mind I float far above the world and look at what is happening below; it looks like a theatre with puppets, which move like driven marionettes. This is what the world looks like to me: mechanical and therefore not attractive at all.

> *I see life as a theater with puppets,
> that move like driven marionettes*

The psychiatrists and therapists have a meeting about my situation and I wait tensely to hear what they have to offer me. When they return with their advice after three weeks, I am very disappointed because it has no depth at all in my eyes: 'I am not allowed to think about death anymore and I have to start dealing with daily things'. What now? I realise that my own current mindset doesn't help me out of the depression either, so I decide to give their suggestions a try - no matter how strange to me they sound.

In the words of Bert Hellinger (the founder of 'family constellations' to which I will return later in this book) I see the advice of the psychiatrists confirmed:
    "We take part in the suffering of humanity. Often the tendency is there to connect with the suffering of mankind. In that situation there is only one solution possible for me, and that is to get involved into something very ordinary, light and everyday. This great suffering you cannot stand as an individual, it is too big. The balance in our soul is very unstable. It goes far beyond our strength to face all that, we cannot bear that. What is finally left is only a silent process. Something

very simple: man, woman, children, play, leisure, happiness and suffering, as it comes. The lightness of the soul has a great power. The very strong is at the same time very light. If you want you can practise this lightness. That happens mainly in the ordinary, daily things." *

The very same day I start with 'ordinary daily things'. I buy wool and start knitting a shawl. Because I am fed up with being thought so young, I go to the hairdresser of the hospital to 'get a haircut to make me look older'. The hairdresser says that she cannot do that, but that it helps if I look angrier.

In the daycare room I sit down with my fellow-patients and I play ping-pong. I tinker during the creative therapy and join in going to the weekly market on a neighbouring square. This last I find terrible; crowds of people shuffling along the stalls.
But I start to like being at the unit more and more. We laugh, cry, drink warm milk in the evening and I realise the humour of the neuroses we all have. In the end I feel it is a pity when the end of my treatment is announced.

I realise the humour of the neuroses we all have

I decide to finish my medical studies 'just for the piece of paper' and to handle the internship very differently. I want to have more fun with fellow students, secretaries, nurses and with other doctors, and not take everything so seriously; I want to live. It takes me quite a bit of effort to fight to get back to my place in my studies, but I succeed. After two months I can slip back in.

---

* Bert Hellinger - *Erkennen wat er is [Acknowledging what is]*

Because I have not said goodbye yet to my psychiatrist in Utrecht, I take the train and go to her to tell her the good news about my regained life-energy. But she interprets my enthusiasm as a manic episode, declares me manic-depressive and prescribes lithium and a physical examination of heart and thyroid to check if those organs can handle the lithium-treatment. I don't agree with her diagnosis and tell her that I won't start this treatment. 'Then wait until you reach the bottom' she responds, so I know that it is good that I have said goodbye to her.

I decide to go on a long cycling-tour in the weeks I have to wait to resume my studies. I buy a racing bike and a book with detailed maps of France, and cycle first to see my former piano teacher in Eersel, with twenty kilos of luggage on the back of my bicycle. I hesitate: do I want to do this on my own? I linger so long in Eersel that it is almost too late to set off. Finally I start out and decide to bike so far that I cannot return home the same day. In the evening I reach Brussels. When I climb the first hill there, the chain of my bicycle comes off and gets sandwiched between the bracket and the frame. With the help of a friendly man I manage to get it loose again. The pride in overcoming this obstacle gives me the power to persevere. I stay in a cheap hotel in Brussels; my journey has begun.

The pride in overcoming the obstacle gives me the power to persevere

---

I have not planned a route, so the next morning I don't know which page of my map-book of France I will open. This makes me realise that I need an orientation point, and I decide to take

Taizé as my first goal. Taizé is a small village of five houses in France level with Switzerland, where a Christian Ecumenical centre is situated on the top of small hill. Young people from all over Europe come together there. You sleep in bunk beds in barracks or in tents. Every morning you talk in a group about subjects such as: "What resources do you have in your life?" / "What gives you vitality?" / "How do you deal with forgiveness?"

At the front of the church, situated in the middle of the ground, orange pieces of cloth are hung and at the side you find tasteful Russian icons of Jesus, Mary and John. Three times a day songs are sung in four-part harmony, simple prayers are recited and in the middle of the service there is a silence of ten minutes. Everybody sits on the floor on a small bench and the young friars - in a white hooded habit - in the aisle. Outside you eat, sing and dance together. It is beautiful to take a walk between the gentle rolling hills and to sit in the small village church with small stained-glass windows. I have gone there once or twice a year since I was twenty; sometimes for a silent retreat of a week.

Through wind and weather I bike in the direction of Taizé. Uplifting music sounds through my Walkman.

I sleep in youth hostels and in a student room in Verdun. Because I cycle about one hundred kilometres per day over quite high hills, my knees become more and more painful each day and by the time I reach Taizé I can hardly walk. I decide to stay there for one week and my knees soon recover.

My second goal is conquering a high pass in Switzerland. It is heavy weather in Switzerland and the pass that I wanted to climb initially is not accessible, because many rocks block the way. Slowly I climb another steep mountain and proudly I conquer the pass.

The descents are most difficult. I learn how to slow down by pumping the brakes. On a steep descent I enter a tunnel, which is pitch-dark because there is a turn in it and daylight cannot enter. My small bicycle light cannot match up with this darkness. There is no cycling track and the cars brush past me. Without light it is very difficult to keep my balance. I ponder that if I am run over in this tunnel, nobody will notice. But, with beating heart, I come out.

Shortly after this, my wheel locks. I seem to have a huge twist in my back wheel, because two spokes have broken from the heavy weight of my luggage. The bicycle repairman orders a new wheel that arrives after three days. As an extra, he checks my handbrakes by squeezing them hard one time, and at that the cable of my front brake breaks, proving that I have got through that tunnel with a very thin cable. I could kiss that man.

In the evening I phone my mother. I feel that she is hiding something from me so I ask her supplementary questions. Then she tells me that her cancer has spread to her lungs. Stricken and immensely sad I sit down on a hill in the dusk and cry. Something beautiful happens then: I suddenly see my mother as a human being and I don't focus on her cancer any more. My medical glasses have dropped off and I feel in contact now with who my mother really is. Because I want to be close to her soon, I cycle even more kilometres per day. When I reach the Netherlands eight days later I am very proud that I have succeeded in accomplishing this whole tour just by bike.

There is so much that has empowered me on this bicycle tour: the use of my physical strength, being in Nature the whole day, repairing my bicycle myself, the connection with people along the way, and being occupied with something totally other than studying.

Using my physical strength and the challenges of my bicycle tour have empowered me

I finish my studies. While I am doing my internship in the hospital, my mother is sitting in the waiting room about to have radiotherapy on her head because the cancer has spread to her brain, something she has always been afraid of. I feel impotent in my white doctor's coat: I cannot save my mother.

My mother wants to get everything possible out of her life. She does everything that for a long, long time she has wanted to do. She gets up at four o'clock in the morning, makes marmalade, learns typing, buys bright dresses with flowers and reads a lot of books about finding strength in oneself and dealing with cancer. At the same time she prepares the house for after she has left the body, so that we will not be lacking anything in the material sense: she buys new curtains and a new washing machine. It is painful for me to see because it announces her departure.

While the tumour in her head makes her so dizzy that she almost falls over, she keeps doing whatever she can: ironing, preparing snacks, cleaning and cooking. The final week she doesn't come downstairs anymore and stays in bed. She can no longer speak and indicates with her fingers what she means. My sisters and I are all at home to care for her together with my father, and in the night we watch over her one by one. One early morning in June, she dies in our presence.

I pass my medical exams and take the Hippocratic Oath, which makes me realise that I don't want always to be focused only on healing at all costs. Death also has to get a place in the whole; a dignified dying, rarely seen in a hospital, where instead treatment is continued until the last moment, often against one's better judgement.

After my studies I fall into a deep hole. My training is finished, while I don't know what to do with it, and I miss my mother. The depression comes back in its full intensity.

I don't know what I have to do with my studies and I miss my mother; the depression comes back

---

Then I decide to go to India for three months, where I hope to find my goal in life. I have already been corresponding with an Indian nun for a while, whom I met in Taizé. She has asked me what I want to do in India and I have sent her some of my ideas.

My sisters accompany me to the airport. My plane is delayed, finally for six hours, because the engines are out of order. My sisters don't know this and have already returned home. I feel a bottomless emptiness inside.

After a long journey I land in Bombay. The person who has come to pick me up - he has been sent by the Indian nun - has been waiting for me for six hours on a stone bench. The bus runs along the slums of Bombay, where girls climb up from the mud to go to school. They wear spotlessly clean school uniforms; a white blouse and a blue dress. Their hair, braided and with bright red ribbons, shines with coconut oil. The corrugated sheets from the roofs look decayed and non-school-going children have smudged faces and tangled hair. Plastic and other kinds of rubbish cover the ground of the slums and the wayside. Seeing so much poverty feels like a shock and I feel the strong impulse to go back to the Netherlands on the next plane.

Depressed, I hoped to find an oasis of rest but the opposite is the case. Seeing people working enormously hard to survive confronts me even more than in the Netherlands with the fact that I don't do anything with my studies. I feel guilty about this and about the fact I don't know what to do with my life.

The hard working people confront me with the fact that I don't know what to do with my life

---

There seems to be a whole programme for me. The nun from Taizé has put into action all the ideas I had sent to her, to the letter. Bye-bye freedom. The programme leads me unwillingly to the most southern tip of India in Tamil Nadu. I feel terribly homesick and want nothing more than to go back to the Netherlands. But when I once tentatively mention this, I see deeply disappointed faces and my guilt prevents me from talking about it again.

In Tamil Nadu I visit a small hospital in the middle of the jungle. I want to see and feel how they work there, because I think - against my better judgement - that working as a doctor in India could be something I want to do with my medical study. In Tamil Nadu it has not rained for three years, because a long time ago thousands of trees were chopped down. The people don't possess a single rupee. There is drought, poverty and sickness. An Indian doctor, a forty year old woman who has been able to study in Italy, operates without gloves and without anesthesia, because there is no money for that. Her fingers move skillfully when she operates, without getting a single drop of blood on her naked hands. Four people sit on the arms and legs of the patient during the operation, to press down the shaking body.

People are waiting in a long queue for the time of consultation: a pregnant woman with a dead baby in her womb, a man with diabetes for whom no insulin is available, a woman with cancer for which no treatment can be given, a girl who is carried inside totally limp because she has taken arsenic, not wanting to be married off - she dies half an hour later. The doctor is a beautiful, good-looking, intelligent woman. She tells me that she has become a Christian nun in order to be able to work as a doctor without having to ask the patients for money. She looks at me with friendly eyes when she asks me how I feel. Then I decide to say it once more: 'I feel homesick.' Finally someone understands; she looks deeply into my eyes and says: 'Then you have to go back; homesickness is terrible. You will return to India one day.' Immediately she gets started with booking my train journey back to Bombay. After the news about my planned journey home, the other - much older - nuns are waiting for me in a large group and start harping on at me: 'Look how bad the situation of our patients is here. Why don't you just stay to do something about it?'

Homesickness is terrible, you have to go back

When I arrive in Bombay again after a long train journey, I hear at the re-booking desk in the airport that I have to wait five days for the first possible flight back. I have come to India with the ideal of not being a tourist here; I wanted to drink tea with the beggars. But the beggars want money from me and are not interested in my tea ceremony. I can't move an inch or people will come up to me: 'Do you want to buy drugs? Change money? See my monkey dancing?' To my great shame I end up in a tourist bus, to get rid of the beggars.

When I cross the street one day with my head down in a very dark mood, I see a boy next to me, walking on all fours because he is handicapped. He has chunks of wood under his hands to protect his palms while walking. Passing me he looks up and calls cheerfully: 'Good morning!' At that, I wake up: good morning! I suddenly see that the sun is shining, hear that joyful music - which still sounded like cats whining the day before - echoing over the street and for a moment I don't know any longer why I was depressed anyhow.

When I am finally able to leave India and stand on an elevated platform at the airport, I see deep down below a beggar dragging her children through the sand to make them look more miserable. I feel that the doctor from Tamil Nadu is right: I will come back here. 'India is life' someone told me once; here you see everything so true and unvarnished.

On a terrace back in the Netherlands one week later, while I am puzzling over what work to do, I suddenly get an idea. Since I seem unable to work it out, I decide to start doing something which has nothing to do with my medical studies. Maybe I will stumble upon my vocation if I don't try so hard anymore to find it.

I sign up at an employment agency and they offer me production work. Now I work with my hands instead of my head and I enjoy seeing what I have done each day in the growing pile of boxes that rises up next to me.

I enjoy working with my hands:
more connection with my body

Besides that I read. Since I was sixteen I have always been looking for books to help me further in my search for 'true life', which makes my mother repeatedly sigh: 'Don't get everything from books.'

When I am reading one day - in a second-hand book shop - the descriptions on the back covers of the psychology books, the text on an orange cover stands out. I don't know the content of the text any more, but I remember how 'true' it was. When I turn the book over at the checkout I get frightened: the book is by Bhagwan Shree Rajneesh, the man of the Rolls Royces. Won't this book be dangerous? I hesitate but the text on the back cover tips the scale and I buy it.

Right away I am deeply touched by the content and I underline almost every sentence. 'Call yourself back thirty-three thousand times a day to the moment of now' really appeals to me and I start practising this immediately. The factory is a great place for it; precisely because the work is so simple - taking ten booklets with the instructions for use of a Philips Shaver from the production line, putting a rubber band around them and putting them in a box - it is very suitable to train myself to remain with my attention in the moment. This gives meaning to my work. My colleagues are surprised that I find so much joy in what I am doing.

Training myself to remain in the moment
gives my work meaning

After a few months however I start increasingly worrying about my future. The work in the factory has been nice for a while, but not for my whole life. My gloominess grows and all energy flows out of me. When my last production-work job ends I ask for unemployment benefit and go in search of therapy.

I don't see psychiatric help as workable any more. During my medical studies I based my hopes of working in the future on psychiatry because I was much more interested in the psyche of man than in somatic diseases. I got high marks for the psychiatric exams but the way of working in this sector disappointed me a lot. While there was a lot of talk about clinical pictures, which were classified using the DSM manual, there was hardly any attention given to the environmental factors or to the social network of the patient, and I missed especially the inclusion of the body in the therapy. Almost everything was treated with medicines, whose violent side effects shocked me.

During my medical studies
I get disappointed in psychiatry

I did an internship at the psychiatry unit of the academic hospital in Utrecht. I was asked to take a psychiatric anamnesis from a twenty year old boy who had been admitted just one week earlier. That boy told me that he read a lot of books about war. His father had experienced the war and he, as a son, was interested in what had moved the Nazis. When reading these books he sometimes had the feeling that he was in the war himself. He asked himself what daily life was all about. Everything seemed to be so futile set against the horrors of the war. I recognized a lot of myself in this boy. Finally he said that he had heard the moon saying something that night, which I also noted down in my anamnesis. I wish I had not done that. When I entered the long corridor of the unit the next morning, the boy zigzagged with flabby legs through the passage. His head was hanging down and his eyes were dull and didn't seem to see anything. He did not recognize me anymore. On the grounds that he had heard the moon speaking they had given him antipsychotic drugs.

My psychiatric lectures were almost exclusively about Freudian psychoanalysis. One day I asked my professor, who told us about all the unhealthy defence mechanisms, what was healthy behaviour. He answered that he didn't know that. Disappointed I put down my pen.

All this has made me decide that I don't want to be occupied with psychiatry or with fighting against sickness, but rather with what promotes health and well-being.

One day I mention in my violin lesson that I am looking for a type of therapy which is not based on analysis from the head. My teacher gives me the phone number of a gestalt therapist who has been very helpful for her. I immediately make an appointment.

Gestalt therapy is a kind of therapy in which you start by listening to your body. Via body signals you stumble upon happenings in the past where you have not been able to complete your natural reaction. Then you work at still completing that unfinished movement. These are exciting sessions, because you never know beforehand what will come up. Often this is anger or sadness, and sometimes I come across enormous rage. Sitting on my knees I express my anger, encouraged by my therapist, by hitting a mattress with a tennis racquet and also by using my voice: or I sit opposite an empty chair on which the imaginary person sits with whom I have difficulties. When I have uttered my grievance or pain to that person, I put myself on the empty chair and answer myself from the perspective of that person. Finally both people are part of myself and that gives me new insights. The therapy helps me to get a better connection with the honesty of my body and also to come more in the moment of now. In that sense it comes together with the book of Bhagwan: 'calling yourself back to the here and now thirty-three thousand times a day.' When I am in the moment I feel alive and freed from continuously following the same thoughts about past or future.

When I am in the moment, I feel alive

I am so happy with this form of therapy that I feel I want to work with it and I sign up for the gestalt therapy training at B.O.L.T: Center for Awareness Development and Learning Therapies. I do two years of the gestalt training and the one-year bodywork training. My father is happy that I do what my heart inspires me to do.

I feel so good now that - besides doing these trainings - I also start teaching nurses in the subjects of anatomy and pathology. The pupils enjoy the lively way I communicate and I enjoy the contact with my students and with other teachers. The only problem is that I don't have enough interest in conventional health care to continue following the developments in it. I feel that I will sell my students short with this in the long run and again the question arises of how to shape the work I really want to do: promoting health and well-being from the inside.

During my gestalt- and bodywork education I practise Zen meditation daily for half an hour. In Zen meditation you sit on a small stool with your open eyes directed to the floor without looking in an active way, by which means you witness everything that is happening inside you: thoughts, feelings, your breath, any sounds you hear as well as silence. It becomes a powerful tool in my life, which I always have with me; in everything that happens I can simply be present and watch. I don't need to identify with those happenings; I am the consciousness that witnesses them. Meditation becomes more important for me than therapy.

However, after three years of Zen meditation I feel that I need a more vivid form of meditation.

Meditation becomes an anchor point in my life

One day I am in a new age bookstore, looking for a book about intimacy. When I haven't found it after searching for more than an hour, I give up and decide to go in search of soothing music instead. On the front of the box with music I find to my surprise a CD with the title 'Intimacy'. It is by Osho, a name I have never heard before. When I listen to the CD I am impressed by the silences between sentences, which give me a deep rest. Later I hear that Osho uses his way of speaking to bring you into a state of meditation; in the silences between the sentences you wait for what he is going to say, meaning no thoughts can arise in your mind. Over the next weeks I buy two books by Osho. With the second book I discover that Osho and Bhagwan are one and the same person.

When I am in Taizé again one month later - it's summer vacation - a woman from Lithuania comes up to me and starts telling me, to my great surprise, about an active Osho meditation which she does in Lithuania together with other women.

She tells me that the Osho Meditations centre is in India, in the city of Pune.

In that moment I feel a powerful ball of energy jumping up in my upper belly. It is a feeling I have never had before and that totally bypasses my mind. Everything comes together: wanting to go back to India someday – searching for a more vivid form of meditation - searching for something that brings me deeper into my *being* - and my dissatisfaction with continuing to teach medical subjects.

---

*I have a feeling I have never had before
and that totally bypasses my mind*

Immediately after my coming back from Taizé I go to a travel agency in Eindhoven and ask where Pune is. The city turns out to be near Bombay on the west coast of India.
Dizzy with excitement I take a seat on a high stool at the counter, take a deep breath and say: "Just book a ticket for after three months - that is the term of notice of my job."

As soon as school starts again I ask my manager for a sabbatical year. This is not possible, so I quit my job and using the savings my parents have put aside for me leave for India for half a year - which finally turns out to be a year. I am thirty-three years old then.

After a long journey I arrive at the meditation centre and one day later I am walking around, like all other meditators, in a long maroon robe. That colour proves to encourage meditation. Osho left his body five years previously but everyone tells me that his energy is present unabated. I am very critical from the start. Because there are so many photos of Osho I am afraid of personal glorification. That proves not to be so. Osho doesn't want people to follow him; rather that everyone becomes more and more themselves.

I find exactly what I am searching for: active meditations, which start with dancing and releasing emotions, along with silence, beautiful Nature and people from all over the world who have come here, just like me, for meditation and their own inner search. The whole day through, meditations are offered in the Buddha Hall: a large marble floor covered with the largest mosquito net in the world. In the morning you can participate in tai chi, yoga or archery. There is a swimming pool, there are tennis courts and in the evening after the evening meditation there is a disco or another activity. The food is delicious, there is a lot of laughter and I feel I can be totally myself here.

Osho wants to bring Zorba the Greek and Buddha together to make life complete and speaks about 'Zorba the Buddha' as the future of the new man.

Also there are therapy groups, therapy trainings, massage trainings, art therapy and many other groups offered by the best therapists in the world.

Everything Osho has said has been recorded on tape and video. When I listen to Osho's words in the morning, I cannot listen for more than ten minutes because what he says touches me so deeply that I can't contain anything more. Tears of deep recognition flow down my face. For the first time in my life I feel understood on the level of my soul.

For the first time in my life I feel understood on the level of my soul

---

Osho understands when you may no longer want to live in this neurotic society. He calls it intelligent if you are considering suicide then, but also indicates that meditation - a way that leads to life - is the alternative. He calls on you to connect with your *being* through meditation, to discover your true nature again, the one with which you were born and which has become overloaded with the rules of society.

I begin a relationship with an Indian man: Paripurna, who works in the meditation centre with a lot of devotion. We laugh a lot, enjoy Nature, meditate, and we cross the hills on his motorbike, singing loudly.

Besides that there is also pain: from the first day he announces that he is polygamous. It is difficult for me to deal with that, even when it contributes to my awareness because I have to examine inside myself again and again what is real love and what is jealousy. I also see that it is not for nothing that I have a relationship with somebody who is polygamous; while I am longing for a monogamous relationship, I am also afraid of a one to one relationship.

After one year in Pune I want to go back to the Netherlands, because my sister who is one year younger than me is about to have her first child. I want to be there for this, even though I am afraid to go home because I will face my conditioning there again. In India, everything is so different from the Netherlands that it doesn't occur to me to start comparing myself with others. So often in the Netherlands this comparison is exactly my undoing.

In India I feel the pressure of my conditioning less

What I have been afraid of happens: I can't find my niche in the Netherlands. What gives me energy, though, is sharing the Osho meditations in the form of the meditation course 'Joy in Daily Life'. In this course I meet people who love meditation just like me and on those Monday evenings I feel just as happy as in Pune.

In India my passion has been touched: it is the sharing of active meditations. But there are still however many unsolved things from my past that pull me down again.

In order to earn money I start working in an asylum in Eindhoven. I feel right from the beginning that this is a wrong choice and that I don't want to work with medicines. After only three months I quit my job, which my colleagues regret because they liked working with me.

I am desperate and feel that there is something very profound inside of me that stops me really living. I want to tackle it extremely thoroughly: twenty-four hours a day. This can be done at psychotherapeutic centre *de Viersprong* in Halsteren.

You can't just join the programme there; you first have to show your motivation. Then there are two initial talks with the main therapist. After that you see how they work during an open day following which you have to write a letter describing your motivation and why you want to participate. My letter is accepted and two months later I can start.

The programme fills the whole day: cognitive therapy, creative therapy, archery, therapy in the swimming pool, chores, cooking together and writing a lot of reports.

After searching for a couple of weeks for my core problem, one morning I get my 'contract' on which I will be working from then on: 'I am no longer mother's dream-princess; I stand on my own feet in the world.'

Pierre, the main therapist, explains how in the past my mother did not want to be alone because of her pain, and wanted to keep me close to her. She made me into her dream-princess by doing and arranging everything for me and by protecting me totally, on the condition that I would stay with her. As a result I have not yet learned to stand on my own feet in the world.

After three months my therapy process at *de Viersprong* is finished, but I don't really feel ready yet to go out into the world.

---

*When I prepare the meditation workshop
all of a sudden I feel my joy in life*

Back home I manage to obtain a free year-long course of career guidance. I join a warm group of eight people; everyone helps and motivates one other. In my individual presentation exercises I always talk about the value of gestalt therapy and meditation. I don't manage to find a good structure, however, to create my work out of this and as the year progresses I slide further and further down into the grey tunnel that I know so well. One day, when in a moment of enthusiasm I am again describing meditation, the group asks me if I would like to give a workshop for them. Right then, I don't feel like doing this at all. But I realise that they have done so much for me that I agree nevertheless.

Back home I start preparing the workshop. I have enough materials from my meditation courses. And then the miracle happens: when I start, all of a sudden I feel my joy again in life.

I make invitations for the workshop out of bright paper, put together a varied programme and feel so much energy that it even causes me fever that night.

The workshop is a success. My group members, who have never meditated before, are excited and ask for a follow-up workshop which I give the next week.

Now I feel that I really want to start sharing meditation and I sign in at the Chamber of Commerce.

Because I still can't get by financially by giving meditations I also start working as a school doctor, and one and a half years later as a company doctor at the *Arbo Unie* in Tilburg. I treat primary school teachers, a target group with whom I am familiar as I come from a teacher's family. They mainly suffer from burn-out, which mostly heralds a change in the way someone lives. Just like depression, burn-out is a signal which offers you the possibility to go for who you really are and for what you really want. It gives me a lot of satisfaction to accompany people in this process.

I also enjoy the contact with my colleagues. Twice a year I can go to the Osho Meditation Centre in Pune, thanks to the fact that my clients have long school holidays. One day my boss asks me if I would like to facilitate meditations on a national level for the companies of the *Arbo Unie*. That feels great to me. However, the terms and conditions of employment take a long time to process, while I feel the longing to go back to India again for a more extended period of time, not at least because I miss my Indian friend. Looking back I regret that I didn't stay in the Netherlands to give shape to this beautiful project: 'the introduction of meditation into the marketplace'.

I resign and in the Osho Meditation Resort in Pune do all the trainings necessary to be able to facilitate each of Osho's Meditative Therapies. Besides that I do the Japanese Face

Massage training and offer from that moment on this rejuvenating and deeply relaxing form of massage in Eindhoven.

One night I have a very symbolic dream. I dream that beside a high old wall there is a huge tree, several hundreds of years old. Overconfident, I climb the tree in order to get over the wall, secretly looking behind me to see if people are following me. But there is no-one. The trunk of the tree forks into two large branches. In an attempt to swing myself over the wall I grab one of them. The branch, however, turns out to be hollow and breaks off. Then the second branch turns out to be hollow too. Suddenly I see that starting from the tree a meandering street of bricks leads to a square in the distance, where a busy market is going on full of colours and noise, laughter and screaming. From that square the road continues further to the spot which I wanted to reach, behind the wall. At that moment I realise that I have to take the way through the 'market place', and that from there I can reach the quiet place behind the wall. I wake up and feel that before starting to share meditations I still want to work in an organization: 'in a market-place'.

I realise that I should not bypass the market-place

I apply for the post of assistant physician at a mental institution in Venraij to utilize my experience with bodywork, gestalt therapy and my medical studies to guide people. I pass the first application round, in the course of which I have pointed out in the job interview that my interest is more in the psyche of man and not so much in the somatic (the physical symptoms). I am therefore greatly surprised when the second round turns out to be a conversation with the institution's nursing home doctor since within the care-plans of the nursing home there is an emphasis on somatic stuff, and I tell the nursing home doctor that it seems like I'm in the wrong movie. He tells me that he would like to work together with me, as well as how beautiful his occupation is, it being a valuable enquiry into what exactly goes on in older people when in them the psyche and the somatic are so closely interwoven. I decide then to take up the offer and ask for a test period of one month with one of the doctors, since by now I have been out of somatic medicine for such a long time. The doctor arranges an internship within two weeks with a young Turkish doctor who cares a lot about older people. I retrieve all my textbooks from the boxes in which I had stored them so as not to see them anymore, and with lots of energy set to studying medicine for the second time.

After the month's training period in Venraij, however, and much to my surprise and that of the doctor who believed he had engaged me, it turns out that I was never in fact employed by the institution.

Nonetheless, the most important thing for me is that I now know that I want to work in this field and so I apply to a nursing home in Eindhoven. They immediately hire me for half a year. After that I find a job in a nursing home in Valkenswaard, where I am mainly employed because of my 'out-of-the-box-thinking'. Then starts my most beautiful time as a doctor: I work with people with dementia, and with very pleasant colleagues. I really feel at home in this nursing home because we work in a holistic way.

---

*Here I really feel at home
because we work in a holistic way*

The work is physically and psychologically demanding: many evening and night shifts; a lot of serious emergencies; having to face the suffering of the patients and their family care givers; the lack of time available for the work of nurses and caretakers in the current system, and more and more working hours because fellow doctors get sick. But at the same time the work is also rewarding and enjoyable: the people are in the 'here-and-now' - I'm deeply touched by the love of the nurses and carers for this target group - and there is a lot of humour, both in the staff and the dementia patients, and I can work in a holistic way there.

Then comes a big shock: a newly appointed interim director tells me, just before I get my fixed contract, that I have to leave. He can't explain why. After fighting it at first, I finally let them buy me out.

Looking back I understand that the flow of my life had to be like this. However beautiful the work in the nursing home has been, it has also swallowed me totally and over the last two years there has been no time left to dedicate myself to the work which is my real passion: facilitating Osho's Active Meditations and the Meditative Therapies, which will soon be complemented with giving family constellations.

I understand that the flow of my life had to be like this

I get unemployment benefits and go first to India for two months to digest everything that has happened. I now know which route I want to take and ask permission from the unemployment benefit institute to write a business plan for starting my own business facilitating Osho Meditations and giving Japanese Therapeutic Facial Massages. After getting the permission I write my business plan within two months. It is approved by the unemployment benefit institute, even though it later turns out to be based excessively on the assumption of co-operation with a centre for people with eating disorders. I make plans to go to the Osho Meditation Centre in Pune (now called 'Osho International Meditation Resort') for two months, to get even more inspiration for my business and to be with my beloved again. I am full of energy and do not yet know that I will enter my (final) depression one week later. I will tell of this in the next chapter.

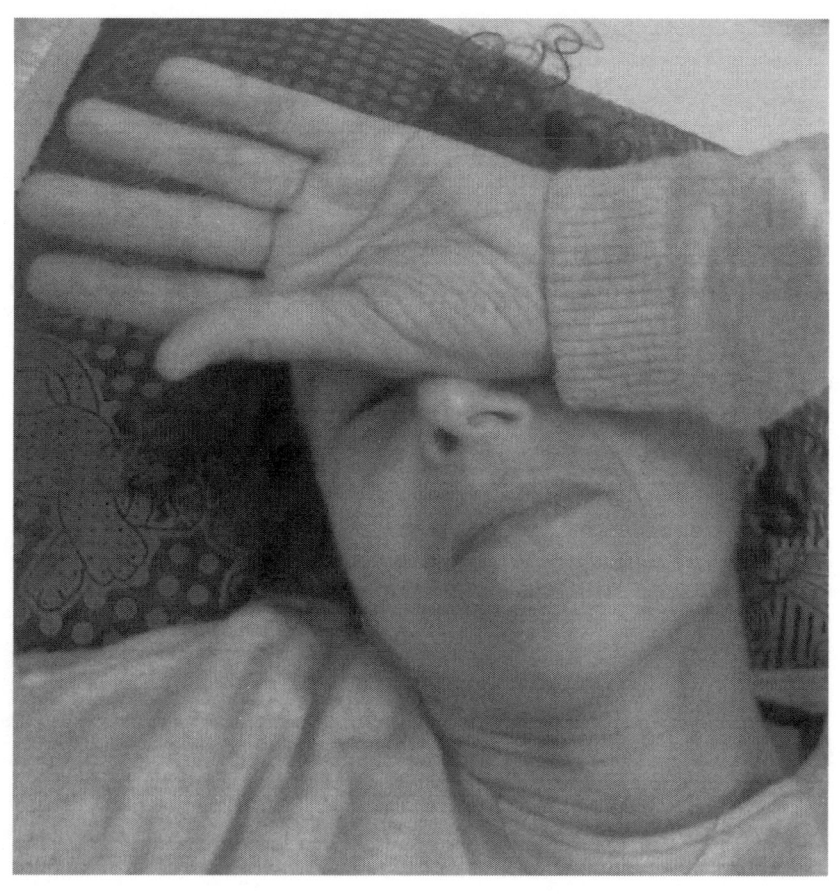

3 MY FINAL DEPRESSION BEGINS

The monster

There it is again. And I had hoped so much never to be as near as this again. A shadow falls over me. I swallow. Sweat comes over me. I feel my throat closing up. I have grown rigid and I feel nauseous. It whispers in my ear and continues going on. The monster of depression. I hate it, because it slowly takes my mind into its possession. Everything it says, hits my head like the stroke of a maul. With each stroke I feel how I become a little smaller. It is back again, while I thought to have turned my back on it forever and I want only one thing: to escape. But how do I do that?*

Janine

Only five days after completing my business plan, I receive a message in my mailbox: the collaboration with the centre for people with eating disorders has been cancelled. With this the backbone of my plan falls away. My hot air balloon speedily shrivels up.

Benumbed, I catch tight hold of my beloved straw, 'India';

---

* Janine - mindblue.nl/ervaringsverhaal *[story of own experience]*

I cling to the inspiration of the meditation centre and especially to being together with my Indian friend. I phone him to say that I will come in just two weeks. Then follows the second blow: he asks me to postpone my arrival because another girlfriend is coming already this month. I had always assumed that I would be a priority for him.

I see the opened jaws of the depression-monster approaching me, slow and inevitable. All life force flows out of me and my body changes into a grey, deflated bag, hardly able to draw itself up. When I look out of the window I see a grey sky without a spark of light and my apartment is reduced to just an empty box.

Inside of me an alarm bell sounds: 'I know this monster and this time it must be possible for me to defeat it.' I give everything I have got to defend myself - body oriented exercises, meditations, positive thinking, texts from Osho - but the depression-animal is stronger.

I understand much better the frustration now of people who think they are cured of cancer and suddenly discover metastases; it is difficult to start the recovery process once again.

Looking back I can see that at that point in time I am not rooted enough in myself to stand up to misfortune, because I am too dependent on my work and on my love relationship.

---

*I am still not rooted enough in myself
to stand up to misfortune*

A new period of depression has started. In the next chapter I describe a day of being depressed.

4 A DAY IN MY DEPRESSION

The only way to die is not dying physically but stopping to move in your heart, your feelings. In the physical sense death does not exist; your soul is eternal and lives on. *

Pamela Kribbe

Every day in my depression passes in almost exactly the same way:

In the morning I don't want to wake up; the night, in which I could submerge all my worries in my sleep, gave me a certain rest which is brutally disturbed by hearing the first birds. Not knowing what to do with this new day I try everything to continue my sleep. I don't succeed. My restlessness increases and changes quickly into panic, which rushes wild and flaming through my chest: 'help, everyone has something to live for and I don't.' Will-less, I whirl around in a bottomless well.

---

* Pamela Kribbe - *Nacht van de Ziel [Dark Night of the Soul]*

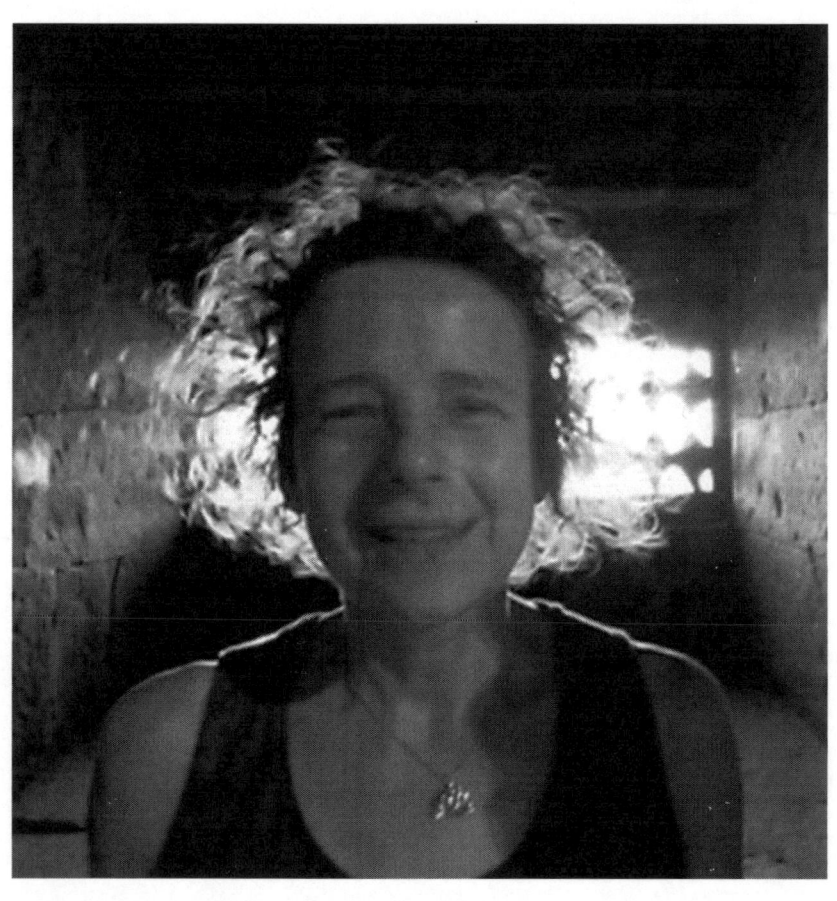

My head makes fierce attempts to find solutions. I call up before my mind's eye my sisters and other people I admire, and imagine to the last detail what they are doing at this moment. The more I become merged into those vivid imaginings, the more my energy is flowing out of me. Still I continue with it; it is as compelling as an addiction. I even mimic with gestures what this or that person must be doing, trying to feel how it is to be really alive. My hope is that when I do what they are doing, I will come into my own flow. Nothing is further from the truth; I float further and further away from myself.

I am hugely jealous of others and this affects my relationships; I cannot be happy with the happiness of another. I feel guilty about the fact that although I breathe, in fact I am living dead.

Although I breathe, in fact I am living dead

After putting off waking-up for one and a half hours, the restlessness drives me out of bed. I am in a hurry because my biological clock is ticking while I still don't know what to do with my life. I put on the clothes from the other day, cover three rice crackers with cheese and set myself down in front of the window at the place where the sun shines on my self-laid wooden floor. Looking at the clouds, which float freely along the blue sky, I relax for a moment.

Then the fear strikes again: everyone is occupied with something except me. I can't bear being alone anymore with this fear and run to one of my sisters, who lives two streets away. I am just in time for coffee. After the second cup I help her with the housework. That help doesn't progress things very fast, because I apply the handbrake in everything I do; I tighten one muscle while pulling my arm or leg to exactly the opposite side with the antagonistic muscle. This way I drop things and make mistakes. There is no energy in what I do, let alone joy. I compare myself continuously with my sister, who is capable of doing so many things in a day.

Still I keep working; to get compliments and to get the feeling that I'm doing something useful. When I cannot stay any longer with this sister I run immediately to my other one, who lives another two streets away. There I repeat the same thing: staying with her as long as possible by helping her.

My next daily walk is towards the supermarket, where every day I buy a bar of dark chocolate that I eat within an hour; I have heard that there is an antidepressant substance in it. After that I eat something from the fridge every half hour; food gives consolation for a few minutes, but is immediately followed by emptiness again.

I cannot stand it for more than an hour in my apartment. In a rush I start walking my restless tour of the neighbourhood. I look through the window of each house to see what others are occupied with; I try to become part of it by watching. But it makes me even more restless because it is so confronting to see what everybody is doing while I am not doing anything. I want to leave all this and drive the car to the *Achelse Kluis*, a monastery just across the Belgian border which is surrounded by a wide heath plain, bordered by woods. Walking along the path right across the plain gives me peace for a little while. But this rest doesn't last long. My concerns about the future pile up as dark clouds in my head.

Back at home I dive into Facebook and gape at the colourful experiences of others. I surf especially to the pages of people who live my dream: facilitating Osho meditations. When I see such a person sitting at the tip of a rock in Bali next to a radiant group photo of the workshop he or she has just finished that day, I feel the bottomless gap that exists between my life sitting on the wooden floor in front of the window and the sparkling life that could be possible.

I lose myself in comparing with others

My hope is set on an oracle: a sentence or saw which will provide me with the decisive indication to a new direction in my life. So about three times a day I consult my tarot cards and the I-Ching, hardly taking time to formulate a question because of my panic. And at the same time everything is a question, because I have lost the connection with myself. I cannot feel which clothes I want to wear, what I want to do, which workshop I want to attend or which answer I will give to someone. Every day I do the same, with the vague hope that one day a solution will come out of the blue. When I open the mailbox, I hope that I will find a letter or parcel that contributes to the solution. But when I open the box I only see its blue varnished bottom with a small rusty edge.

Regularly I send panic mails to my sisters and to friends from Pune: 'What should I do to get out of this situation? How do you live? Do you have a suggestion for me?' Their first answer is often helpful and empathetic. But two to three emails later I notice from their comments that they are tired of getting my cries for help presented in exactly the same terms again and again. The live contacts I have with the few people I still meet grow worse, too.

Because I feel hurt so quickly, almost every meeting ends in a conflict. There's not much kindness in me; jealousy sets the tone; I blame the other that he or she lives their life and I don't. I notice how I leave a trail of destruction behind me, which plummets my self-image even further.

I notice, how I leave a trail of destruction behind me

One of my sisters points out regularly that I behave like a victim. That is difficult for me to hear, although I know that she is right. 'Being a victim is the most cunning form of revenge', Bert Hellinger writes in his book *Ordnungen der Liebe [Orders of Love]*. Looking back I can see that this is true: I take revenge on everyone who is not depressed and on my parents who I feel should have done things differently. Unconsciously I convey: 'look how unhappy I am'. I have heard it said that underneath depression lie suppressed anger and sadness, but in my emotionless state this is hard to believe.

The sentence 'I want to be dead' is often humming in my head without me making active plans for suicide. In a passive way I defy fate by carelessly crossing the road.

I am looking continuously for a way to overcome my depression. Every day I browse the internet looking for therapies, workshops and trainings, which promise a bright future. Sometimes I see that the 'saviour' workshop will start that very evening in a distant city and in panic I grab together my nightgown, toiletries, train map and purse. My inner handbrake however stops the movement at the last minute and

I unpack my bag again. Not being able to choose between two workshops which overlap each other in time becomes a fixed pattern. For days or weeks I remain in the dilemma: workshop A or workshop B? The corners of my tarot cards curl because of their frequent use in an attempt to make the choice, and in my wooden floor appear little holes because of frantically tossing the I-Ching coins. When I finally start workshop A, I go on imagining how it would be if I had chosen workshop B, so that I am never really present in what I have 'chosen'.

In the evening I feel better. Now I know that everybody has come home and is not so active any more, just like me. On my tour through the neighbourhood I see people sprawled out on the sofa in front of the television. Now I can also allow myself to rest. Because it is more bearable for me now, I stay up late to read or to watch television.

The night promises to be a pleasant anesthesia of the torment of the day and I hope that it will last as long as possible.

Where everything in me seems to have come to a full stop, underneath life still appears to be flowing. To speak with Osho's words: 'Life is a continuous flow, nothing remains'. This flow creates a change in my depression which I will describe in the next chapter.

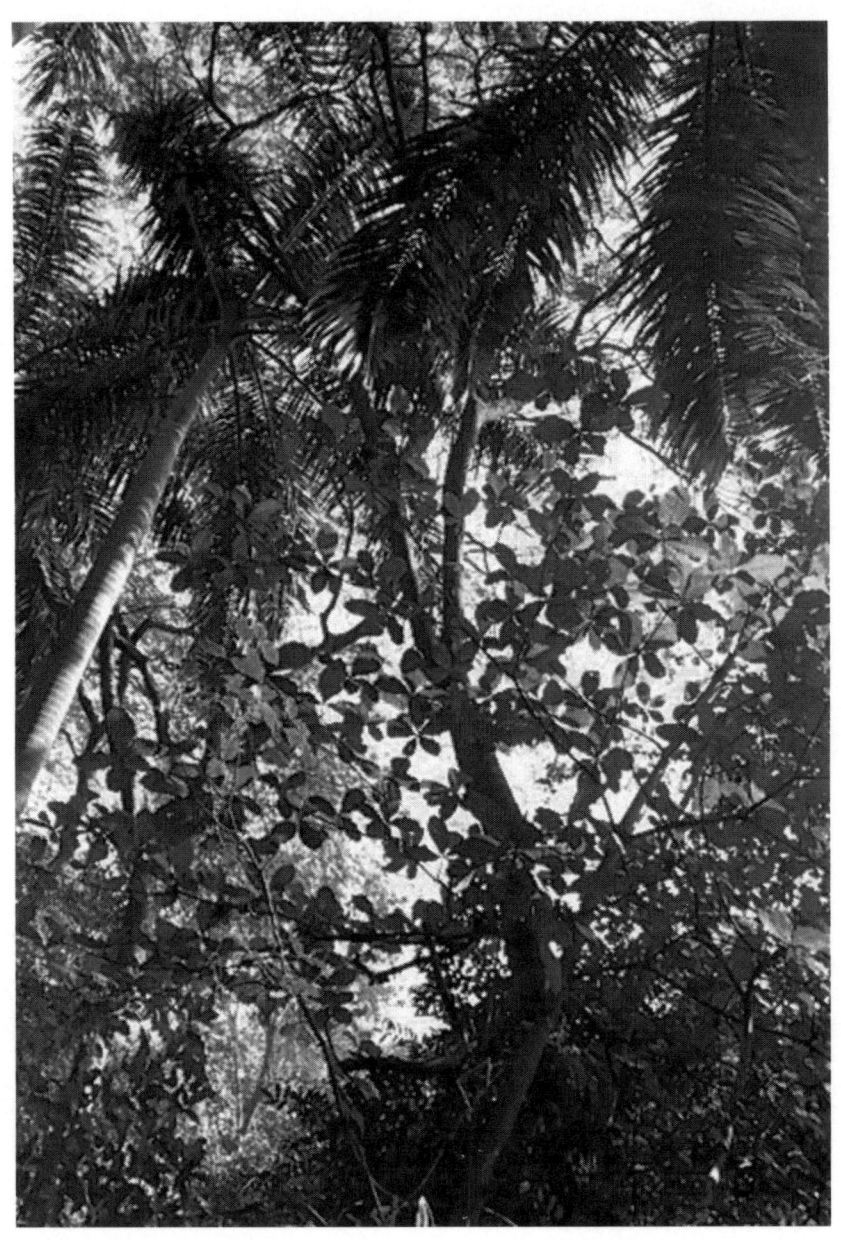

5 THE TURNING POINT IN MY DEPRESSION

"And I make it an absolutely necessary point that there is nothing more therapeutic than love. Technique can help, but the real miracle happens through love." *

Osho

My sister tells me that her friend has had a psychological examination - which was covered by her health insurance - in the psychotherapeutic centre *de Viersprong* in Halsteren. This examination seems to me a good opportunity to see which therapy will help me best. I get the required referral letter from my family doctor. The examination consists of four parts: first, an encounter with a psychologist – then filling out a long questionnaire – next, an interview to determine my character structure and finally a talk with a psychologist who reports the final conclusion of the examination. The advice to me is: Schema Therapy.

---

* Osho - *The Great Pilgrimage: From Here to Here # 14*

Schema Therapy

It is up to me to find a place where this form of therapy is offered. I find it at *de Grijze Generaal* of the *GGz* (psychological health care) in Eindhoven. It's a therapy which lasts more than one year, either two or three days a week. I am shocked on hearing the duration; one year is so long! I elect three days per week because I need structure, so the more time I am there the better.

---

*I need structure,
so the more often I have therapy, the better*

A reference from the family doctor is once more needed. Immediately I make an appointment to get it and the family doctor promises me to send the reference straight away. When I phone the *Ggz* three months later to ask when it's my turn to start the therapy, however, the reference seems never to have arrived. I have to wait for another six months.

In the meantime, though, I am offered to be taken on now by the main therapist, to which I immediately say 'yes'. One week later I'm sitting on the edge of my seat in the consulting room of Ed; a tall middle-aged man with a friendly, somewhat aloof face. I am in a hurry because my depression has already lasted so long. Agitated, I tell him as many details of my hopeless situation as possible and ventilate my great expectation of this therapy. Ed however leans back in his chair further and further and, although he continues to be friendly and laughing he makes it immediately clear to me that he cannot guarantee the success of this therapy and that he doubts whether it will catch on with me anyhow, because I have had so much therapy and still I am depressed. He doesn't see why this process would suddenly help me now. He also thinks that my patterns might have got too engrained in me because of my age. Moreover, he thinks that I won't really fit with the people who will be with me in the group because we have very different backgrounds; for example, they don't have any interest in meditation.

The small trace of courage that I had left sinks down to my boots. I feel now that the success of a therapy will not depend so much on the form of the therapy, but on me.

I feel that the success of a therapy will not depend so much on the form of therapy, but on me

---

To go through a therapy does not automatically guarantee success. Despite so many valuable things having been handed to me in the many workshops, groups and therapies that I've had in my life, I have not been able to integrate them into my life so far.

Although before the conversation with Ed I was still wondering if I would start this kind of therapy, which is so cognitive - coming from the head - I feel now that I want to fight to be allowed to take part in it. I convince Ed that I will do everything possible to make this journey successful and he puts me on the waiting list.

Outside the swing-doors of the *Grijze Generaal* I am struck again by doubt: 'Modita, you don't want this, do you? Aren't you one of the people in favour of emotional body work and gestalt therapy? Such a cognitive therapy doesn't mean anything to you, does it?' Being a patient of the *GGz* means for most of the people in the outside world that you are at least a little bit crazy, which is hard for my ego.

When three months later I have the introductory talk with Anja - one of the therapists of my future therapy group -, my doubts disappear. Not so much because of what she says, but because of who she is. I feel an instant click with her. She greets me as an equal and looks at me with friendly, shining eyes. We take a seat at one of the tables, which are arranged in a square. Anja turns out to have been in India a lot, just like me, where she has participated in several retreats. When I tell her how many doubts I've had about this form of therapy, she says that it's good to be critical and that this therapy is not appropriate for everyone. I appreciate her honesty, although something in me would have preferred her to say: 'This therapy is definitely going to help you.' Then I could have pushed away my own responsibility.

When I express all the worst case scenarios I have about my future and the sad reflections on my past, she brings me back - from a strong inner determination - again and again to: 'being with what is; feeling without judgment what is here in the moment'. This appeals to me; it comes together with the message of Osho and with my own longing.

The purpose of the schema therapy is that you start investigating in detail what life patterns (schemes) you are involved in and why. Then you examine step by step what you can do to free yourself from this. The therapy is divided into blocks, ranging from half an hour to an hour and a half. There are verbal blocks: these consist of cognitive therapy (in which you gain more insight into the schemes you are using), sharing rounds (sharing about what you are going through in your daily life, and in which the group members and the therapist can give feedback) and one hour per week in which you examine your home, work and leisure situation. There are also non-verbal blocks: psychomotor therapy in a gym (where you work with everything that you encounter through games and in physical contact with others) and creative therapy (in which you express your feelings and life themes with materials like paint, clay, fabric, wood or soapstone).

Every week one of the group members organises a block in which he or she talks about a hobby or interest - giving the others a taste of that - or organises a game, a movie or a walk. All in all we have six therapists for all these different blocks.

The nonverbal therapy forms appeal to me most. They are in line with what I have experienced as so valuable in gestalt therapy, emotional bodywork and the workshops and meditative therapies in Pune.

The nonverbal therapy forms - psychomotor therapy and creative therapy - appeal to me most

---

My group consists of eight people, who are all in different phases of the therapy. The longest in the group is already there for more than a year. The most recently arrived participant is there just a month.

A week after the conversation with Anja I meet with the group. When I enter for the second time the bare group room - they don't make it cosy on purpose so that you don't want to stay there - I quickly check if I feel a click with somebody and heave a sigh of relief; everyone seems to be nice. I introduce myself comprehensively, being as open as possible about myself because I think this will speed up my process.

Looking back it appears that the members of my group are startled by my verbose introduction; they fear that my verbal presence may inhibit them getting a word in during the therapy blocks. They also turn out to be not exclusively nice. Even from the very first Monday a struggle for time and attention starts between me and the young woman who is the longest in the group. I also get into trouble with her that first week, because she is so helpful that it suffocates me.

I miss meditation as part of the therapy. It is there, but for no more than five minutes per week in the form of a guided visualization. We conjure up in ourselves a safe place, where we can always return if we want to feel secure and at ease. For me it is the white plastic chair on the edge of the swimming pool of the Osho Meditation Center in Pune, under trees which shine in the morning light. I miss Pune very much but know that I need to be here at the moment.

I miss meditation as part of the therapy

Ed was right that I would find it very difficult most people in the group having such different backgrounds to me. They come from a very different environment and don't have to do much with meditation. I experience their being-different as threatening.

The purpose of the schema therapy is that you start investigating in detail what life patterns (*schemas*) you are involved in and why.

In the first three months I discover my main schemes:
- social isolation
- entanglement
- failing and inferiority

Social Isolation

My schema of 'social isolation ' is immediately evident: apart from with my sisters I barely hang out with anyone, out of shame that I have no work or children (even though I have consciously chosen the latter) and therefore don't share anything meaningful with the world. Besides that, I envy others and stay away from them so as not to be confronted too much with the sparkling lives they lead. On one hand I feel inferior but on the other hand, I feel more special than others; two sides of the same coin.

I discover in the cognitive therapy that I have cut off my emotions so as not to feel the lonely vulnerable child in me. I have been hiding behind a distant, sometimes haughty guardian, who approaches everything from the mind.

Another defence mechanism that I have developed is to dissociate from the established order and give the impulsive, undisciplined child in me free play.

It is hard to really acknowledge and accept the vulnerable child in me, because this fragile child is even more afraid to be hurt when it shows itself. I notice however, that I have much more the feeling of really being alive if I dare to be vulnerable than when I armour myself and lose the connection with myself and with others.

I discover that I am much more alive
if I dare to be vulnerable

After three months, as well as the group therapy I also get individual sessions with psychomotor therapist Theo. Theo is a quiet, sensitive man with sharp eyes, who accurately observes someone's smallest movements. Just drawing conclusions is something he doesn't do. The questions he asks me give me a lot of space, and when I have told him something, he often closes his eyes to absorb it totally and to really understand it.

In one of these sessions Theo and I are back-to-back and very close together, a small distance between us. We close the gap by moving our backs very slowly together until we are leaning against one another, and then move away from each other again - all this without talking. The intention is that I perceive in detail everything I feel. Theo himself does this also. Then we share our experiences.

It is scary as hell for me. I want to do it 'right', but do not know what is 'right' in this case. I feel the first touch. Theo is very careful. Because of fear my sturdy part takes over; I will just show that I am not afraid and that this is a piece of cake for me. I lean back heavily and had hoped to get more pressure in return from Theo. Immediately afterwards I'm afraid that I'm too demanding and ask too much, or that I am too dependent. I'm scared to death of being rejected and concerned that Theo will break the contact. So I decide quickly to be the one who ends the contact. Pretty soon I release myself from his back. When the connection is broken I feel very lonely and sad. I associate the loss of contact with the loss of my twin sister in the womb. When we share our experiences, Theo indicates that he felt contact with me for a moment and regretted that just when he wanted to rest in that contact, I was already gone.

It feels good that I have experienced so much in just two minutes. It feels like being alive and not depressed, because I *feel*. I find it nice that Theo would have liked to have connected rather longer, but I also find it threatening that he feels something different to me throughout the whole exercise. I recognize that I always hope that someone else is exactly the same as me and that I often become angry with others when they appear to be different. I don't know whether this has to do with missing my twin sister or with the symbiosis with my mother, or maybe with both. I am learning that having contact has to do with resting in my own body and enjoying this, by which I allow the other to do the same and to also be him- or herself, and that the exchange happens in the contact area of our being-different. It is very scary for me to enter into this. I have to dare then to be alone with myself, with my own feelings. This ends the symbiosis I have had with my mother so long. Only when I accept the being-different of the other, can I really meet him or her.

Only when I accept the being-different of the other, can I really meet him or her

---

After a couple of sessions with Theo I find more and more rest and a basis in myself, from where I can connect with the other person without losing myself.

First in the therapy group and later also outside the group, I practise with this. It takes trial and error. The members of my group give me positive reflections in their feedback. Little by little I start enjoying the new experiences between me and the other, even when I face difficulties with it; because now I see these difficulties as a challenge.

Entanglement

The schema 'entanglement' is a tough and difficult one, which already exists at my birth: I start being entangled with my mother when I feel how much pain she carries inside. I identify with her and try to carry her pain by proxy, which in the first place is not possible; it is the pride of a child to assume such power. My entanglement with her means I hardly learn to feel myself or to develop my own point of view.

As a child I have the illusion that I can carry the pain of my mother for her

---

In the family I feel very responsible for maintaining harmony and take a mediating position, in which I don't ask enough attention for my own emotional needs. In conflicts I twist and turn to make sure that the others feel good, without asking myself what I feel or need myself.

This entanglement becomes a pattern; I get entangled with my sisters and with the people of the workshops and trainings I follow. It's almost impossible for me not to get entangled.

When for example at a party Mrs. Babble says something, and I see that Mr. Silent also tries to speak, I ask Mr. Silent a question, so that he can also be included. Then I feel guilty that I have interrupted Mrs. Babble. Being then so occupied with apologizing to Mrs. Babble I don't even hear Mr. Silent's answer to the question I have asked him. I've also seen already that Mrs. Critical is irritated by all this, so from that moment on I am also trying to appease Mrs. Critical. In this way I lose a lot of energy.

The entanglement also gives me something positive, however. My efforts give me the feeling that I matter to all these people; I make sure that everyone gets a word in and feels comfortable. The price I pay for it however is too high; I lose the connection with myself and don't follow my own feelings anymore.

It takes me a lot of effort to step out of this schema. For this I need the courage to stand alone and in myself. Meditation helps me, even though meditation is very difficult during my depressions. When I do an active Osho meditation (about which I will speak more, later in this book) at home, it gives me a good feeling. By meditating I feel an anchor point in myself, on which I can always fall back.

In the years after the schema therapy I am increasingly able to untangle the intertwining-knot. I recognize earlier when I am entering this schema and can decide to stay out of it. More and more I lead my own life, in which I set my limits and no longer need to give meaning to my life by entangling with others.

Failing and Inferiority

I felt as a child that my parents had high expectations of me, even though I never heard them say it aloud (they always told me: 'What matters is that you are happy and not what you do'). I tried to meet their expectations through studying hard. In my depression it feels like a failure that I don't do anything with the study, in which they have invested so much of their time and money.

My feeling of having failed is reinforced by my psychological problems, which make me feel like a burden to my parents. My mother is worried every day during the six years that I have anorexia and she is sad when I go to school with a minimal breakfast in my stomach, and my father is also sad when he sees that I feel so unhappy. Nonetheless, I feel that my father has always been proud of me despite my depressions.

A few years before he dies he says that he is happy that his daughters have all ended up doing something else than what he had in mind.

By slowly making connection with the vulnerable child in me I feel how uncomfortable and left out I have felt in high school, for which I have tried to compensate by focusing totally on my study. In the schema therapy group I notice that this experience has made me more on guard; when there is a conflict with one of the group members I easily take my refuge in attacking.

I also see now that I have partly hidden behind spirituality to avoid facing earthly life (in the sense of making contact with others, making my home cosy, finding work), and to evade making any mistakes. Besides that, I have raised my future ideals more and more, which has totally paralyzed me. In the therapy I start making small, achievable steps, which sets me in motion and gives me the feeling that I am alive. It gives me peace when I look back on such a step and wonder what I might want to do differently next time.

Small achievable steps set me in motion

I learn to shift my focus from 'having to do something great' to 'enjoying something small'. Even when a small project flows into a disappointment, it is satisfying anyhow, because I feel enriched by having had one more experience. It gives me more and more fun to learn something new and to experience new things and it increases the positive image of myself.

My experience with the Schema Therapy

The good thing about the schema therapy is that I have a daily structure again. Every morning I have a place to go to on my bicycle. I also meet other people without having to make an effort to look for company. It's liberating that I am among people now who are not from my own family; I can share things without feeling the emotional ballast of what my feelings trigger in family members. I have real coffee breaks again, and listening to the experiences of my group members makes my world grow wider.

After a few weeks I am not so much concerned with the differences between me and the other anymore, but start to see the similarities.

Previously I have looked down on the everyday things of life. Now I experience how precious it is to share my daily habits and worries with the members of my group. It is healing for me that they sympathize and actively share thoughts with me on how I can handle the difficulties that arise in my daily life. More and more I open myself to their advice and I am moved by the sincere support I get. It also feels nice to me to think of things with them and that it is appreciated.

The therapy process does not pass without some friction, however. There is even a lot of it: some group members really get my back up and then I am sitting behind my small table boiling with anger. In this setting I cannot escape the seemingly minor things that affect me so much.

It is super-confronting for me to sit behind my table in that grey room in the building of the *GGz* day in and day out, often without much progress. Sometimes I don't even see any progress at all, although the other members of my group don't agree.

Certainly a hundred times I indicate that I will stop in a week's time. I want to go to the Osho Meditation Centre in India then, where I always feel good. No one forces me to stay. Nor does my beloved therapist Anja. She consistently says: "It's always good to remain critical." And yet: I remain and there is not a single day that I don't attend. I stay because I have no alternative. Only in the years following the therapy do I see clearly what I have learned here; I have summarized it above in the description of each schema.

After I have been one year in therapy, I complain about the fact that I don't have a focus in my life. A group member recommends I make a focus-stone in the creative therapy block. That idea appeals to me. I carve out of pink soapstone a small thin rock that rests on a two millimetre base - steep, pointed and perky. The light twinkles, sparkling in the soft pink stone. I put it gently before me on the table and all of a sudden there is my focus. I decide on the spot to do the three-week long 'Osho Art Therapy Training' in the Spanish Basque country: painting as a therapy with Osho as a source of inspiration, led by the Japanese artist Meera Hashimoto. For the first time I am able to choose again.

There is all of a sudden my focus:
the Art Therapy Training of Meera Hashimoto

---

the Art Therapy Training

Meera Hashimoto, a Japanese artist, has developed Osho Art Therapy: painting as therapy. You rediscover in this training the creativity in yourself that has always been present, but which has often been suppressed by your upbringing and by the education system. Osho meditations (about which I say more later in this book) are an important part of this form of therapy. In the Art Therapy Training you also learn how to guide others in this process. For this, going through your own process is essential.

I have already had the opportunity a few times to help in this training when Meera offered it in Pune. As a 'helper' then I used to put in an enormous amount of work: mixing the paint, fitting plastic on the marble floor on which we paint outside, carrying the wooden boards which serve as the blotting-pad of the papers we paint on, arranging the group room and much more. As a helper I was allowed to join the training for free. It has always brought me a lot: liveliness, connection with myself and with others and with creativity. Since I feel that I have not come out of my depression totally yet despite the schema therapy, this is why I hope that this training will bring me back to life again.

Because Meera knows that I am emotionally stuck, I am only allowed now to do her training as a participant, so that I can do the process totally, only for myself.

I have a lot of respect for Meera: she lives what she teaches; she goes deep in her meditation, is merged into her own painting and is very committed to reviving creativity in others. She works from a space of love, respect and equality. With her I feel very clear how much healing happens through love and respect.

With Meera I feel very clear how much healing happens through love and respect

---

The training starts in two weeks, which means that if I want to participate, I need to stop with my schema therapy earlier than planned. My therapists agree with that. Two weeks later I complete my therapy and three days after that I'm sitting on the plane to Bilbao. On three buses I travel further to Amalurra; a beautiful centre in the rolling hills of the Basque country run by a community of people who meditate together every day. Here I will follow the Art Therapy Training with twenty-five participants and ten helpers, who come from all over the world.

At the centre is a large restaurant where we are served the best food three times a day. The therapy room, which the people of Amalurra have built themselves, looks like a temple, with walls which almost completely consist of windows so that you can see Nature all around. I sleep with two other people in a room, which is not easy because one of them snores like a charm.

When we sit in a circle on the first morning together with Meera, I tell the group in the introduction round that I'm depressed and that I find myself socially isolated.

Meera looks at me with penetrating eyes and says: 'So just inquire how you bring yourself into that isolation - why don't people feel safe with you - why do they run away from you - what is the cause of your creating an unloving atmosphere around you. This you can't fix in one day; keep exploring'.

Bang, that hits me like an arrow. It is a tap with the well-known Zen stick of Meera. Not 'poor-you-why-are-you-so-down-and-lonely?' It's totally up to me, to examine what exactly I am doing. I realise: who can look into this matter except me alone? I am my own researcher and at the same time my own research subject. Because she has the confidence that I can do this, I feel, despite - or maybe thanks to - the tough message, respected by Meera.

From that moment on I take responsibility for myself. Deep down I have always felt that I was avoiding this responsibility. I always looked up to people who carried their own responsibility and who were therefore mature. I have always stuck to the conviction that this is not within my reach and I have always been looking for excuses in the past to justify this. Now I realise that I can still start this very moment to take full responsibility for all my actions.

I realise that I can still start this very moment to take full responsibility

---

With each contact I now observe myself: what exactly do I do in a contact? How do I make myself victim? What comparison do I make of myself with the other? When don't I ask the other how he or she feels but am only concerned with myself? When do I make my own problem the most important thing in the world? How do I avoid contact? How do I give up trying to connect with the sentence in my head: 'I can't manage anyhow?'

This self-examination becomes the first important pillar in this training for my healing and growth.

The second pillar is the 'Osho Dynamic Meditation'. It is a physically and emotionally intense meditation, which we do early in the morning and about which I say more, later in this book.

The third pillar of my healing is family constellations. Also to this I come back later.

After the morning meditation we paint - interrupted by the delicious meals and a siesta - from early morning until late at night on large handmade sheets of paper on the floor.

We give space to the inner child to express itself completely. We make contact with each other by painting in each other's drawing, which makes me feel how the other enriches my creativity and my life, and how I add something to the life of the other. We learn to say 'no' to what the other person does in our painting, and to say 'yes' to the contribution of the other and above all: to say 'yes' to life. We meet our inner critic and learn to sell our painting (our creativity): to really stand up for it. In the section 'self-portrait' we sit behind mirrors on the floor and meet our parents through our eyes; the right eye is connected with the father and the left eye with the mother. Meera teaches us, and lets us feel, that you can only be creative when you have a good connection with your mother. Family constellations (to which I return later in this book) help to see that which stands in the way of that connection. By seeing this obstacle it resolves.

In the last week we descend to a little creek that flows between the soft lush greenery of trees and creepers. We paint there for hours, each on his or her own spot, inviting exuberant Nature onto our paper.

Dancing is an essential part of the training. We dance our painting and paint our dance.

---

*You can only be creative
when you have a good connection with your mother*

In this training I regain my life. Meera sees it and asks me if I want to help her in India once again in the training she will give in Poona in half a year. Out of pure joy my arms fly around her neck. She looks at me and says: 'And now never go back into depression again.' I know this will never happen; something in me has been completely cleaned up and I feel anchored in myself; light and full of colours. I will continue with meditation, connecting with my body, with getting deeper roots in the earth and with sharing what has taken me out of the depression. I will share it with those who, just like me, want to get back their life through awareness. Now the sharing of meditation no longer arises from an attitude of being a meditation teacher, but from my guts, from a deep lived experience.

Six months later I help Meera in the Art Therapy Training in India. I mix the paint, rub the floor, help the participants with what they need and participate in painting myself.

Then, one year later, suddenly the news of the death of Meera reaches me. She has died in a diving accident; she has become one with the ocean of life - the lively ocean, about which she talked so much and which she lived. I can hardly believe it and know at the same time: Meera will always remain; dancing and sparkling. She is everywhere now. The people who have always worked with her continue her trainings in Pune and in many other places in the world. You will find the programme on her website: www.meera.de.

Thank you Meera!

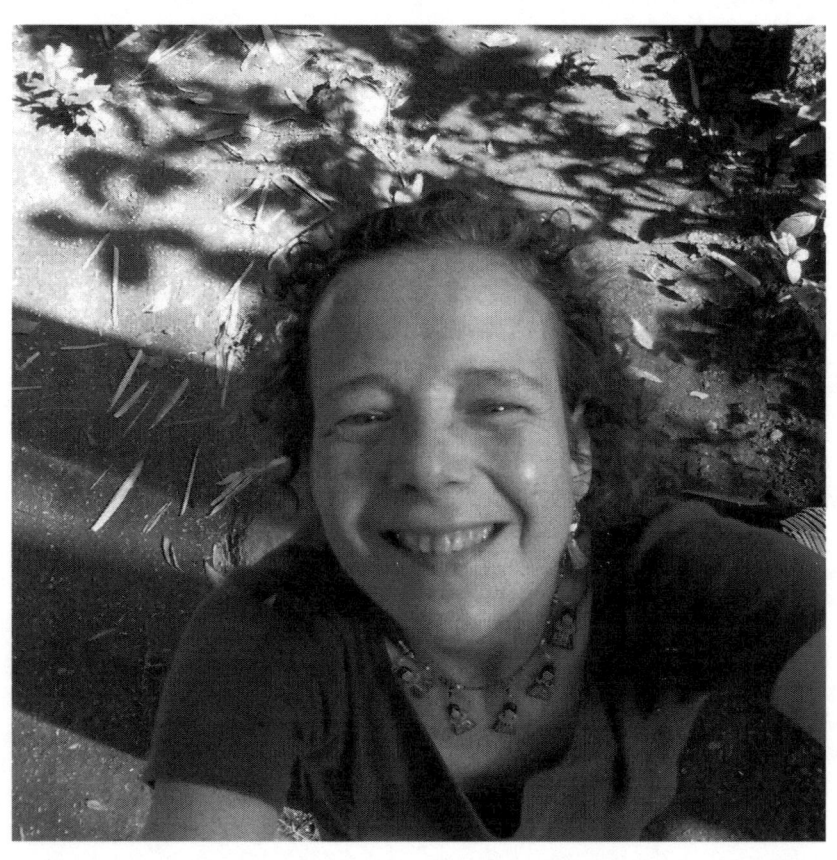

6 A DAY IN MY HAPPY LIFE

*Thank You, o God, I want to thank You
that I can thank*

Evangelical song bundle 168

With the help of the guidelines which I will describe in this book, I have definitively come out of my depression.

At the end of my personal story I describe a day in my happy life right now.

I am already awake before six o'clock. The awakening summer light shines softly through the salmon-coloured curtains and the first birds are chirping. Silent and grateful I listen to the twinkling song with deep silences in between.

I stretch myself and jump out of bed. I am looking forward to start the new day. First I do my stretching exercises; I move each joint separately, so that the waste which has accumulated during the night can be released. It gives a nice, fluid feeling. Then follows my ritual of thanking all family members - both the living and the dead - and all the organs and parts of my body. In this way I start the day with gratitude for my body and for everyone around me.

I am looking forward to the new day and feel grateful

Then I do the Osho Dynamic meditation, which I will describe later in this book. In this meditation I come to life totally through the intense breathing in the first stage, releasing my emotions in the second stage, tapping into my power in the third stage and enjoying the silence of fifteen minutes in the fourth stage, in which nothing in me moves. I start loving those fifteen minutes of silence in this meditation. It is so special not to do anything at all during a quarter of an hour; I only am and I wait only for myself. The silence also helps me to be patient throughout the whole day with everything that happens. In the fifth and last stage of the meditation I dance the new day. I experience it as a gift to be able to dance life already so early in the day.

Then I take a shower and prepare my breakfast: porridge with nuts, cranberries and dried apricots. I am looking forward to eat outside on my balcony. This I do all year round, even in winter, except when it rains, when instead I'm sitting before my open door. Under my balcony are the colourful gardens of the two sides of the street, with lush trees, flowers and many birds. In fact I have the largest garden of Eindhoven, without having to work on it. On my balcony I have sown wild plants and there's a lot which grows up from the underlying gardens:

grapes from my downstairs neighbour, roses from my other downstairs neighbour and the wisteria of the neighbour next to me. This makes me feel like a princess.

After my breakfast I take my daily piece of dark chocolate and start the work that is my passion: writing this book and preparing the meditations which I facilitate. Besides that I give a number of Japanese Therapeutic Face massages every week, through which I enjoy the silent connection I have with the person who receives this refined form of massage. It is so beautiful to see the peaceful face of the client after the massage and to feel the silence and the space of *being* that has arisen in him or her. I feel rich with this work.

I nourish myself with healthy food and notice the effect that it has on my body; I have become much more energetic and also more calm, not least because I cut out coffee a long time ago.

Because I get up so early I go to sleep for one hour in the afternoon. I sleep very deep then, and when I wake up, I have fresh energy again for the rest of the day. In this way I have two days in just one.

I enjoy the people I meet, where we inspire each other. I prefer to chat with girlfriends while having dinner in the city. My sisters and I make contact as equals, because I have my own life now and also because my jealousy doesn't disrupt our relationship anymore. I can enjoy it now when others are happy. In the meditations which I facilitate and the massages that I give I enjoy hearing what people experience and to see the growth that everyone is going through in his or her life.

Because I had a heel spur years ago, the consequent underdevelopment of the muscles of my right leg has led to an overburdening of my right knee. For ten months I exercise every day for one hour to strengthen my thigh muscles and I walk half an hour per day. Although it is a lot of practice over a long time, I'm happy to be able to do this for my body. Once when I was depressed I wished that something would happen which would literally prevent me moving forward anymore, because that fitted with how I felt. So I brought it on myself. Now I am able to do all this exercising to heal myself, and working on my leg muscles feels like working on being able to stand on my own feet. The daily walk adds much to my life. Every day I enjoy the Nature so close to my house; the sunlight on the leaves, the birds, the murmuring water of a small creek and the people who do sports in the park in their bright clothes. I see the flowers and tall trees with whimsical trunks, and I enjoy now seeing others being active because I enjoy what I do myself.

I feel blissful and appreciate this all the more because I have known the grey desert of depression; because there was a period in which I thought I would never be able to say: 'I am happy'.

I value my happiness all the more because I know how it is to be depressed

---

I attend trainings now which fit with the work I do: courses in family constellations, trauma work and Zen counselling. I fly to other countries to get the best trainings possible. In my daily life I practise what I have learnt in those trainings, because in working with people it is of primary importance to be in balance yourself.

After eight o'clock in the evening I don't touch the computer anymore and don't look at television either because I want to come to rest before going to sleep. I walk a lot, work further on my mandala, read a book and take a shower sometimes. After having pampered my body with a nourishing cream I go to sleep with a satisfied feeling, looking forward to the next day.

I can digest set-backs and emotions more easily now because I know how to use the resources both inside and outside myself. I have a rhythm in my day, where I do what I love to do and can now be both alone and with others. Stress and relaxation I alternate with each other. And above all: I feel grateful. My gratitude I want to share in the form of writing this book.

I can digest set-backs more easily now because I can use my resources

---

My way out of depression has begun at the moment that I took the helm into my own hands. This is the subject of the next chapter.

Part 2

Taking the Helm
into your Own Hands

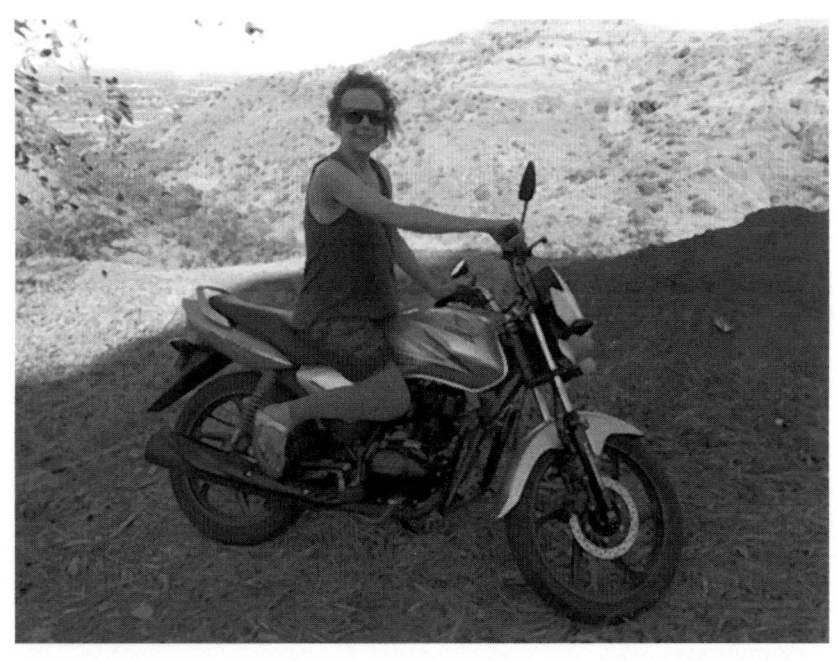

7 THE VALUE OF TAKING RESPONSIBILITY FOR YOURSELF

Existence is a deep freedom. If you want to be in suffering, be in suffering. If you want to be in bliss, be in bliss. It is your own choice. But it is too much for our minds to think that everything is our choice because then we become responsible. If you come to think that you are the cause of your suffering, then you will feel very bad. It always feels better to make someone else the cause of your suffering. But remember, if someone else is the cause of your suffering, you can never become free. Then there is no liberation. But if you are the cause of your suffering, then liberation is within your hands; you can do something and change it.*

Osho

In my depression I send an email to Pavitra Wolf Matthews: 'Help me, I can't get out of my depression.' Pavitra is a wise woman, rooted in herself. For several years I have had craniosacral sessions from her every few months. She has always believed in my potential, however depressed I was, and has often said that she is eager to know what work I will eventually be doing. Several years ago she moved to Sweden.

---

* Osho - *The Supreme Doctrine #9*

Her reply to my request for help is unsparing: 'That you feel unhappy for such a long time means that you have not done your homework.'

---

*That you feel so unhappy
is because you have not done your homework*

Poof, that hits me. Not, 'Oh, how sad for you, what can I do for you?'

Her words stay with me, mostly because I feel that she speaks from her own experience. It must be that she is doing her own homework. I start to realise that there is no royal road to freedom from my depression: that there most probably will not be any single redemptive therapy session or workshop which will change my whole life. The homework as she means it must have to do with practising.

Then what to practise? In fact, I know the answer to this question: I have not fully integrated into my life what I've been given in my many training courses, workshops and trainings. I have always expected, more or less, that solutions come from outside and what I have learnt will automatically stay with me. I have thought emerging from my depression would bring me effortlessly into a harmonious and stable condition which I wouldn't need to work to maintain. Until this moment I have assumed that people like Pavitra have something which I don't have, that they are already rooted, stable and balanced naturally.

I have always felt that deep down I don't carry responsibility for myself and thus I am not mature, and have brought up all kinds of excuses from my past for this, like: 'I have not been able to lead my own life because I wanted to carry the pain of my mother, I have been overprotected by my parents,

I have not learnt from my parents to stand firmly in society.' In fact, I refuse to give up my child-position because I am angry that I did not get what I wanted from my parents. I still want to get it and therefore stay small in the psychological sense. I ask others (friends, sisters, therapists) in different - often indirect - ways to carry the responsibility for me.

Meera Hashimoto opens my eyes in the Art Therapy Training to how stubborn a child can be in his or her opinion. When the child suffers pain, they sink their teeth into it and start seeing everything through lenses coloured by what has happened in that painful moment. When we become adults we often still see through those coloured lenses and don't see the reality of the whole situation: that our parents are also just ordinary people with their own imperfections, people who are sometimes tired and for whom bringing up a child is not easy, and who also carry all kinds of unprocessed things from the past.

The child in us sees through coloured lenses by which we lose sight of reality

Bert Hellinger (founder of family constellations, to which I return in a later chapter) describes in the book *Acknowledging What Is* that you cannot force the process of maturing. I cite: "Those are things that develop naturally in a family. A child is very closely bound in the beginning, but then the room to move enlarges. Later, if the person has taken everything that the family has to offer and treasures it appropriately, then things proceed smoothly, without effort. The individual needn't strive to become an adult; he or she *is an adult*. Whatever I have to intend to do is not something I really want, or I wouldn't need the resolve to push myself. The intention itself is an indication that something is missing, that there's something I haven't taken, or there's something that must be brought into order. When such demands are raised, I know that there's something that has yet to be completed. Then I try to help the client to correct and complete whatever is missing, or to release it."

With me it has literally been like this. The family constellations in Meera Hashimoto's training enable me to receive from my parents, and this nourishes me. From that moment I am willing to carry the responsibility for myself and to open the tool box in which everything that has helped me in my life is available; physical exercise, meditations, family constellations, walking in Nature, healthy eating, the words of Osho, connecting with others and all the insights I have gained about myself. I am determined to keep using all this, in order to never go back in the direction of depression again.

---

*From the moment I can receive from my parents,
I am ready to carry the responsibility for myself*

When somebody asks Osho if therapy groups bring you to your natural self, Osho answers:

"No, that is not the purpose. The purpose is simply to make you aware of where you are, what you have done to yourself - what harm you have been doing continuously and you are still doing. What wounds you are creating in your being. On each of the wounds is your signature - that is the purpose of the group, to make you alert about your signature. That it is signed by you, that nobody else has been doing it. That all the chains that you have around yourself are created by you. That the prison you live in is your own work. Nobody is doing it to you. Seeing it, that 'I am creating my own prison,' how long can you go on creating it? If you want to live in the prison, that's another matter - but nobody ever wants to live in the prison. People live because they think, 'Others are creating the prisons, what can we do?' They always go on throwing the responsibility on somebody else. Down the ages, they have found new and different devices, but the purpose remains the same: throw the responsibility on somebody else.

The purpose of the therapy group is to make you aware of where you are, what you have done to yourself

---

"The group therapy is to make you aware that neither God is responsible nor society is responsible nor your parents are responsible. If there is anybody who is responsible it is you. A group process is a hammering of this simple fact - that it is you who are responsible. And this hammering has a great significance. Because once you understand that 'This is me, I myself am doing wrong to myself,' the doors open. Then there is hope. Then something is possible.

"Revolution is possible through responsibility, individual responsibility. You can transmute; you can drop those old patterns. They are not your destiny. But if you accept them as your destiny they become your destiny. It is all a question of whether to support them or not.

"And I am not saying that parents have not done something to you, remember. And I am not saying that the society has not done anything to you - I am not saying that either. The society has done much to you, the parents have done much to you, the education and the priest, they have done much to you. But, still, the ultimate key is in your hands. You can drop it, you can drop the whole conditioning. Whatsoever they have done, you can erase it - because your consciousness at the deepest core always remains free. That is the purpose of a therapy group, to bring this truth home: that you are responsible.

"'Responsibility' is the most important word in a group-therapy process. Nobody wants to take the responsibility, because it hurts. Just to see the point, 'I am the cause of my misery,' hurts very much. If somebody else is the cause, one can accept it, one is helpless. But if I am the cause of my misery, it hurts. It goes against the ego, it goes against the pride.

"That's why group therapy is a difficult process, hard. You want to escape - from encounter, from Tao, from primal therapy, you want to escape. Why do you want to escape? Because you have always believed that you are perfectly right, you are perfectly good - others have been doing harm to you.

"Now the whole thing has to be changed; you have to put everything upside-down. Nobody is doing any harm to you. And if they are doing any harm, it is through your co-operation.

"So finally you are responsible, you have chosen it. You say, 'My husband is doing harm to me' - but you have chosen this husband, in fact, only so that he can do harm to you. You wanted to be harmed and that's why you have chosen this husband, this wife."*

When I am the cause of my misery, it hurts

To be able to take responsibility, consciousness is needed. When in a depressed state, there can be a strong tendency to

---

* Osho - *Take it Easy #12*

benumb yourself in order to escape the desolation you feel. Then the temptation to start taking antidepressants can be strong, although in fact they reduce the very consciousness that you so much need to get out of the depression. Besides that they don't help in most cases. This is the subject of the next chapter.

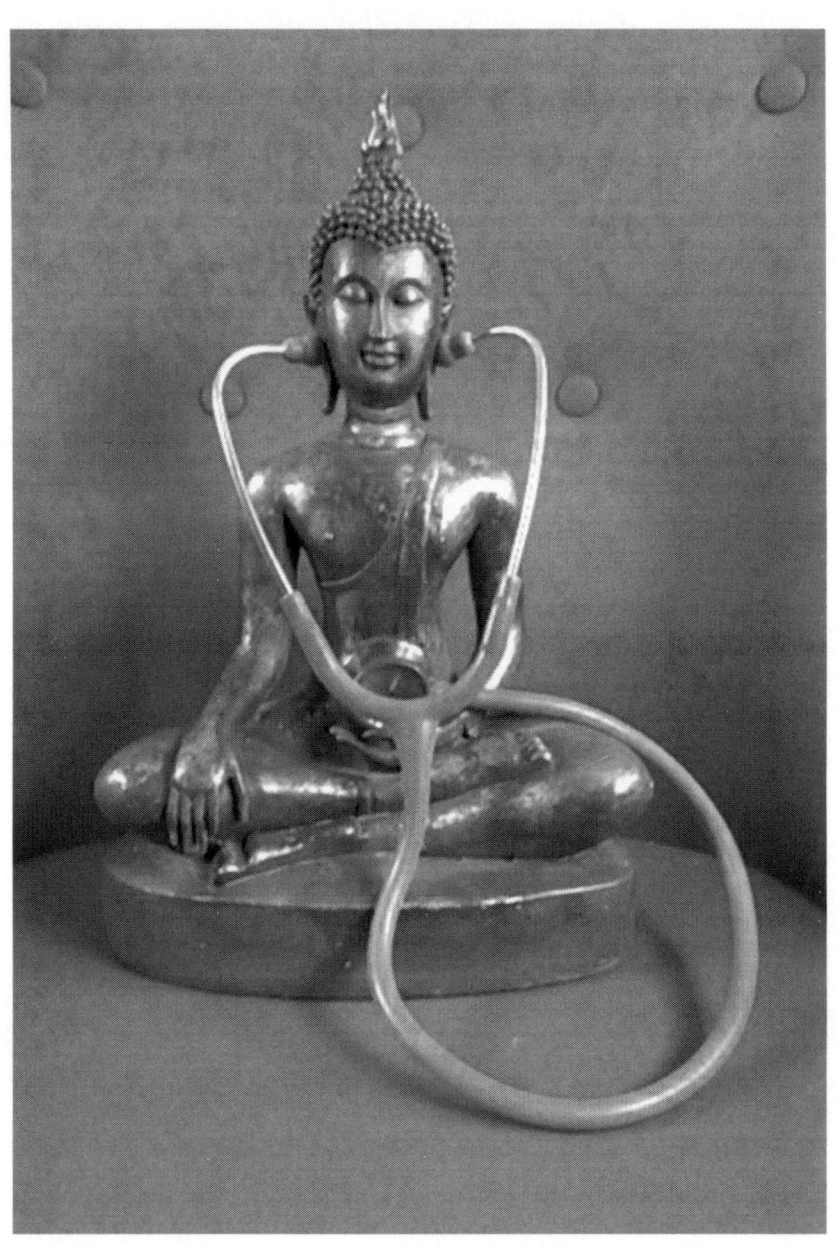

8 THE ILLUSION OF ANTIDEPRESSANTS

Antidepressants

No clue about what I want
I have no power at all
For this feeling I have a pill
Which tones down my feelings
Pleasant and safe
But is this now my life's purpose

*from: Hartenkreet [Cry of the Heart]**

Desperately I ask my family doctor for advice when I fall into one of my depressions. She acknowledges my distress and refers me to the best psychiatrist she knows. With her mediation I am able to see him within three weeks. He receives me lovingly and in the beginning he listens very well.

Every three weeks now I sit in his waiting room and look at the desolate buildings across the street. I hate the Netherlands: everything is grey, grizzled, tight, boring, made of concrete and colourless. I don't even want to have to look at these

---

* *Hartenkreet Schrijver [Cry of the Heart Writer]*: B, 03-02-2013

disgusting boxes of bricks in which people live, mechanically doing their thing. I miss India with all its colours, the life on the street, women carrying a jar on their head, people sitting by the side of the road, just to look around. I miss the bullock carts, the people with a plastic bag over their head when it is raining, the school children - barefoot or walking in flip flops - the girls with coconut oil in their black hair and red ribbons in their braids. I miss the coloured houses, yellow, pink, light green and blue, and the painted trucks decorated with garlands around the windows and with a shoe, dangling from the rear bumper, with the words above: 'horn please'.

In addition to the interviews with the psychiatrist I get the opportunity to take part in a second type of therapy and I express my preference for emotional bodywork. The psychiatric team however decides otherwise. In their opinion I would need support for my daily routine and they link me to a social worker. I am angry about this, and indicate that I have never had a problem wanting to do my own laundry, prepare my meals or go out for a walk so long as I have felt passion, and in fact have taken pleasure in doing all these kinds of things: that is, when I have found meaning in my life. It is now because this passion is missing that the daily things make no sense at all to me.

The daily things make no sense at all to me, because I miss meaning in my life

---

I remember my first visit to my Chinese friend, whom I met a few years ago at my factory job. I had barely arrived in the long hallway of her apartment when she suddenly opened a small cupboard and said, "Look, on the top shelf is my food and on the bottom shelf the toilet paper. That's what I do:

eat and shit. I want more in life!" Blown away, I gave her my gift: a pink piggy bank. Looking back, it's quite appropriate: 'Oink': eating and shitting and hollow inside.

My psychiatrist says that I am just applying the handbrake all the time, which according to him is caused by my anxiety. Although he isn't someone who prescribes medicines by default, he still recommends that I now mute the anxiety with citalopram. He assures me that a low dose of 10 milligrams a day will hardly have any side effects and that any such will be gone after a few weeks.

For weeks I resist the very idea. I don't want that chemical junk in my body and also don't want to depend on it. How will I still be able to follow what is happening inside of me when my feelings and consciousness are dulled? I am also afraid to become even more of a zombie than I am already by now.

Still, it goes on haunting me: what if that psychiatrist were right and I were able to take steps in my life all of a sudden because I was less fearful, even if that were thanks to an artificial substance? Finally I give in, mentioning that I will stop taking the pills the moment my meditation (even though it doesn't amount to much at that moment) begins to suffer under the medication.

Still it is with quite some resistance I drag myself to the pharmacy, and when I finally look at the medicine boxes lying on top of my kitchen cupboard, it feels like a defeat.

The side effects are already there after two hours. A cork-dry mouth, blurred vision, dizziness, and the feeling that my head is cluttered with cotton wool. Emotionally, something inside of me is muted, which may be perceived as 'peace' by some people. But it is not a real peace; it's more like a kind of anesthetic. I start sitting under the tree of that anesthetic like a shapeless sack of potatoes. But by the side of the sack of potatoes is still sitting an anxious quivering creature. It has become smaller, but it is unmistakably there; ready to stand up when the anesthesia has worn out.

You see? I had already been expecting this. How can a medicine solve everything which is hidden underneath a depression? It is a pure fraud. My meditation doesn't work at all anymore.

How can a medicine solve everything which is hidden underneath a depression?

The drug certainly mutes my jealousy of people who are happy but it gives way to total indifference. I don't care anymore how someone else feels. It's like I've become a paper doll, a kind of wallpaper in the background of life.

The side effects don't decrease either. After three weeks they are still present, undiminished, and what is worse: the moments of happiness which - looking back - still had been there, are totally gone. These were moments of happiness which lasted half an hour, or one hour: when I went to my sister for coffee, and was cosy sitting with her at the kitchen table with the red-and-white checkered tablecloth, or when I went for a walk with my other sister. Now nothing can tempt me anymore. My family doctor tells me very honestly that as long as I continue citalopram any moments of happiness that disappear will not return. She suggests another antidepressant, but I don't want to take any of them. I stop taking the drug. Fortunately I can do this straightaway, because the dose was so low and because I didn't use the citalopram for longer than three weeks.

Natural recovery from depression

Often a natural recovery from a depression occurs within three months. It used to be considered normal that you were gloomy for a few weeks after you had ended a relationship, lost your job or a loved one had died. In the latest version of the DSM manual which is used by psychiatrists, now only two weeks of lethargy are considered to be a depression. The criteria used in this manual are also very vague, with the result that one doctor makes a completely different diagnosis from another. A person can often be prescribed antidepressants at their first appointment with the doctor or psychiatrist, without any examination into how they could deal - possibly with the guidance of a therapist - with what is happening in their life.

Antidepressants often have an anesthetic effect, so you can no longer clearly see what feelings are hidden under the depression. This means you don't feel the need so strongly to begin processing them, with the help for example of therapy or meditation. All your unresolved issues are kept anesthetized by the medication.

The pharmaceutical industry has a lot of influence on doctors, even though they often do not realise it. Antidepressants were put on the market when sedatives did not make enough money. Because depression was diagnosed so often, the pharmaceutical industry started researching chemical treatments for depression. These studies showed that antidepressants did not work in light or mild depressions. These research results were hidden by the pharmaceutical industry.

Antidepressants don't work for light and mild depressions

Peter Gøtzsche - Danish internist and professor of clinical research - has reviewed and examined most of the studies done in the field of antidepressants. He describes his findings in the book *Deadly Psychiatry and Organized Denial*. What these studies show is that the functioning of the brain is much more complex than we are led to believe by the theory of 'the serotonin deficit in depression', and also that the side effects of antidepressants can be serious and even fatal, while the drugs are also highly addictive.

The idea that depression is caused by a deficiency of serotonin loses ground

---

In my training as a doctor I have blindly trusted what was stated about antidepressants in my text books, not knowing that there was a lot of information not based on truth. Many doctors are hardly aware of the side effects of antidepressants, even if they are mentioned in the package leaflets. The pharmaceutical industry has obscured many of the serious side effects.

Peter Breggin, Danish psychiatrist, comes to the same conclusions as Peter Gøtzsche. He has also studied and written about research in the field of antidepressants. You can listen to interviews with him on YouTube.

Serotonin levels in the body can be increased without medication, simply by following the right diet. I will tell you more about this in the chapter on nutrition.

Side effects of antidepressants

When you disturb the serotonin metabolism by taking antidepressants, this has consequences throughout the whole body;

these are the side effects. These side effects are usually much more harmful than any possible efficacy the antidepressants might have. Only in severe depressions can the benefits of the medication sometimes be greater than the disadvantages, and at the end of this chapter I describe how you can distinguish such a depression from a mild one.

Side effects of antidepressants are declining ability to think and to learn, declining memory, flattening of the emotions, emotional instability, drowsiness, being easily irritated, having tantrums and the decline of sexual feelings. Because of the numbing effect of antidepressants, it is much more difficult to experience pure emotions, clear consciousness, liveliness, creativity and meaning. You are less able to deal with the difficulties of daily life. It also becomes more difficult to enter into and maintain social contact.

The ability to love, to be creative and to experience spirituality also decreases. When you phase out the medicines all these qualities come back again.

Antidepressants diminish the ability to love and to experience creativity and spirituality

Higher doses of antidepressants can give rise to a great restlessness and the urge to self-harm. Some people have a gene anomaly which can cause the concentration of the drug in the blood to be much higher than intended, with even more side effects as a result.

A serious side effect that Peter Gøtzsche found in the search results is the tendency to suicide; the number of suicide attempts is doubled by antidepressants. The drugs can also create a strong urge to rob someone else of life. Someone who has never before had aggressive tendencies can murder a family member after taking the medication. When such a person phases out the antidepressants, he gets back his normal personality.

Suicidal thoughts, manslaughter and self-harm are side effects of antidepressants.

Withdrawal symptoms after stopping antidepressants

The antidepressants increase the amount of serotonin between the nerve cells. The body's response is to make the body less sensitive to serotonin. The result of this is that when you phase out the medication (you should never stop all of a sudden, because that is life-threatening) the body experiences a lack of serotonin. The withdrawal symptoms that arise then are severe nightmares, sweating, trembling, anxiety, dizziness, being unsteady on the feet, the feeling of electric shocks in the head, fever, flu symptoms, mood changes, nausea, phobias, facial twitches, a generalized sensation of drunkenness and also suicidal thoughts and depression.

These withdrawal symptoms can still occur years after the medication has been phased out.

Antidepressants disturb the balance in the brain

One of the withdrawal symptoms is depression. When this symptom occurs, the doctor, the psychiatrist and also the client often mistakenly think that this means that the client needs to continue antidepressant medication. As a result, hundreds of thousands of people are wrongly taking antidepressants.

Peter Gøtzsche indicates that it is easy to distinguish whether the occurrence of the depression is the result of phasing out the medicines or whether it is an actual depression. If the depression is the result of withdrawal, it occurs very quickly after the medication is phased out and the symptoms immediately disappear when you take the full dose again. In the case of a real depression, on the other hand, it will take weeks after resuming the full dose before the symptoms begin to reduce and you feel better.

Depression is a withdrawal symptom that can occur when an antidepressant is phased out

Phasing out antidepressants

It is very dangerous to stop taking the medicines abruptly. You can get so extremely agitated that you start to behave in either suicidal or murderously violent ways.

Stopping taking antidepressants abruptly is very dangerous. They have to be phased out gradually

So slowly phasing out is necessary. You can do this best under the guidance of a doctor, psychologist or health worker who is open to it and who has experience with the process.

Unfortunately, very few doctors have this knowledge and experience. Often a lot of perseverance is needed to get rid of antidepressants. It can take more than a year, or even several years, depending on how long you have been taking them.

It is a myth that antidepressants reduce the incidence of depression returning: on the contrary, they even increase this possibility.

Antidepressants in severe depressions

I have one clear example from my doctor's practice in the nursing home for dementia patients, in which a woman with a severe depression was helped by antidepressants. All day long she was sitting on the bed in her room. She couldn't pick her life up any more after her husband died. The only thing she could say was: 'He is not here.' She ate almost nothing and was a fervent chain-smoker. She didn't go anywhere anymore and hardly slept. When I started working in her department she had already been taking an antidepressant for years. Consulting a psychiatrist I phased out her old antidepressant and prescribed an antidepressant from another category. Then the miracle happened: she came back to the common living room again, went to the village, accompanied by a fellow-worker to buy three sets of new clothes and chatted and joked with the staff and fellow residents. She still missed her husband, but it didn't paralyse her any more.

So in some cases of severe depression an antidepressant can be of help to make a new start again.

The difference between a mild and a severe depression is that in a mild depression you can be cheered up for a while by something (such as a visit from your children or a friend), after which you drop back again into depression when it's over, while in a major depression there are no circumstances at all by which your mood can be improved.

Building up alternatives for antidepressants

What I recommend if you are using antidepressants already, is to first use the guidelines from this book before phasing out the medicines. It is not for nothing you are using the drugs, so there is something in you that you want to protect. It is necessary to develop some tools first, which you can use to meet the challenges that confront you.

Phasing out an antidepressant becomes easier when you first develop tools in yourself to meet the challenges of life

---

When Veeresh - who has founded the therapeutic meditation- and training-centre *Humaniversity* in Egmond aan Zee - tells Osho that he wants first to help drug addicts to kick drugs before teaching them meditation, Osho says that he has first to teach them meditation before taking the drugs away from them, or else he will create a great emptiness in them not replaced by anything else, and this is inhuman.

The first guideline I'm offering to help you come out of depression is 'saying Yes'. This is what the next chapter is about.

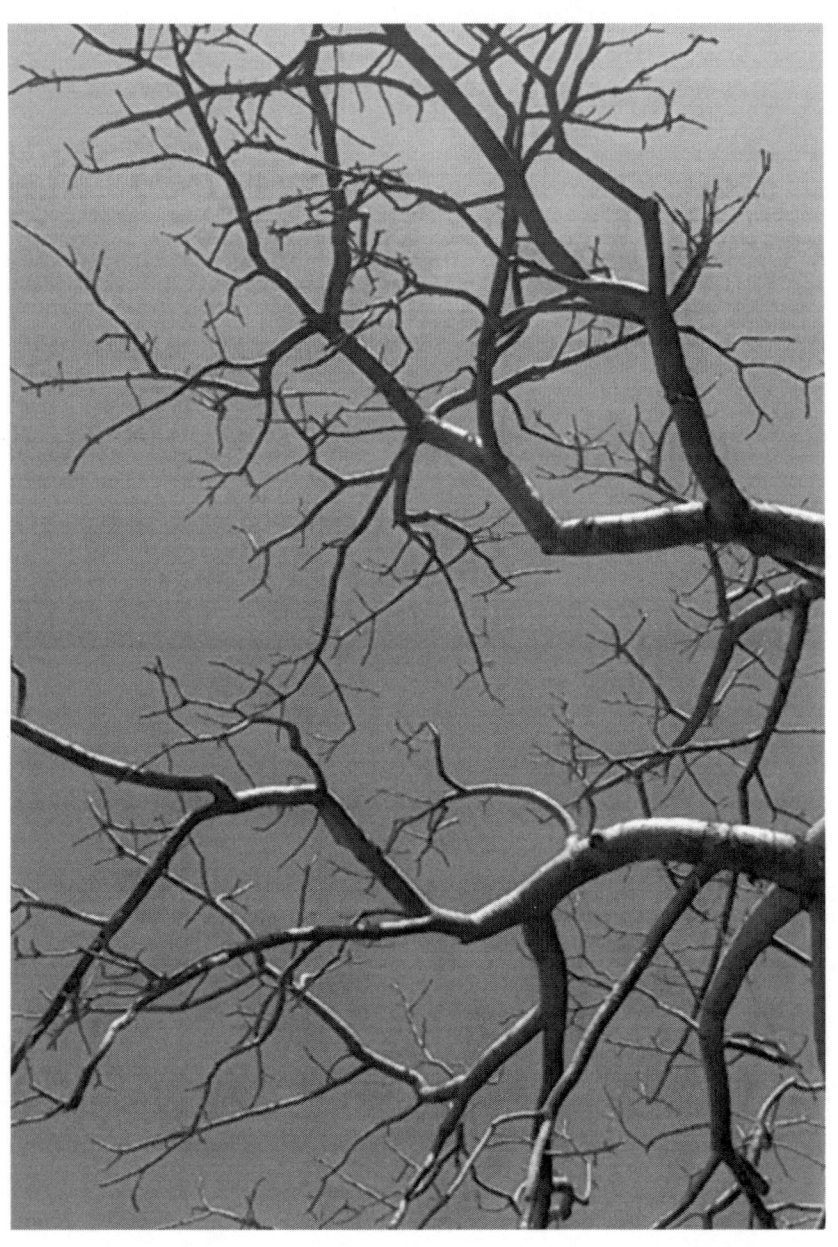

9 SAYING 'YES' IS OPENING YOURSELF TO LIFE

When you say an unreserved Yes to life, life says a resounding Yes to you. *

Pamela Kribbe

During my depressions I have a 'no' to life. Many times a day the phrase 'I want to die' is running around inside my head. Because I stick to 'no', no space can arise for a 'yes'. 'Yes' is life. 'No' is death; a dead death.

My 'no' shows in many ways. When I clean something in my little apartment, I only half-do it, in a careless, sloppy way. I do the same with shopping for food, taking a shower and washing my clothes.

My 'no' is also extended to contact with others. If they do

---

*   Pamela Kribbe, *Dark Night of the Soul*

something for me, I reject it; it is never good enough. When somebody says that he loves me, I don't believe it and assume that it is only said out of pity. When someone gives me something, I find myself not worth enough to receive it and think that the gift is given because the other finds me pathetic. When someone spends time with me I complain that she leaves so soon and think that she leaves because she doesn't like me.

All the time in the background is: 'I'm not worth it - there is not enough for me - people don't like me anyway - people don't mean what they give, they just pretend.' And the more I think like this, the more I see it confirmed.

I feel that I leave a trail of destruction behind me because of this negative attitude, and that lowers my self-esteem even more.

Because of this a lot of quarrels and conflicts arise, especially with the people I love the most. I see it happening but do not know how to change it.

The way to the Light

In their book *Spirituele Verdieping [Spiritual Deepening]* Fons Delnooz and Patricia Martinot describe the choice you have at any time of the day; to move more to the light or towards the dark. 'The light contributes to joy, love, light, strength, truth, sincerity, purity, honesty and beauty. The dark is that which denies love.'*

We are much more strongly attracted by the darkness. To a large extent this is because we have often been brought up by people (parents, teachers, grandfathers, grandmothers,

---

* Fons Delnooz and Patricia Martinot - *Spirituele Verdieping [Spiritual Deepening]*

priests) who were in darkness themselves. If as children we felt happy, we would not belong to them anymore. Soon we started realising that we were loved more when we were sad or gloomy than when we were happy. As a child you need the support of your parents. As an adult courage is needed to get out of this pattern of 'being unhappy for the sake of others'; the courage to dare to stand alone and to move to the light.

---

*Courage is needed to dare to stand alone
and move to the light*

You can apply moving to the light to everything. When you eat something: does this food give you a good feeling in your body or does it take you to darkness? Is this what you really want to eat and do you want to eat it at this place, or rather in a different spot? When you wake up: do you really want to stay in bed? Does your body feel comfortable that way or does it want to move, even though you may not know in what direction? Do you really want to talk with this person, or don't you want to at all? Would you like to see this TV programme, or do you feel that watching it brings you to darkness?

You can feel it in the body, because the body is the most honest; much more honest than your head. Your head is manipulated by your educators, parents, teachers, priests, club leaders. It is an art to teach yourself to observe very accurately. In the beginning you may not manage to sense it, because often you have unlearned it at a very young age. You have unlearned it, because you were taught to fit into society, to be able to operate in your culture (which is also necessary of course). For that you have paid a price: you had to start suppressing a lot of feelings.

It may seem that it takes something big to come to the light, but Delnooz and Martinot emphasise that it's just little things, very small sparkles of light, which if you put them together form the way from darkness to light.

It's the little light sparkles which - if you put them together - form the way from darkness to light

---

What Delnooz and Martinot describe really appeals to me and I start to practise. I notice that I need to be fully conscious for the movement to the light. Many times a day I ask myself now: does this thought, act or body posture bring me more to light or more to darkness?

When I have a thought I observe what it does to me. I feel it in my body and with my energy. If I notice that a thought pulls me down, I consciously choose to think something which gives me a more positive feeling. In this way I don't suppress the negative thoughts, but examine carefully in myself how these thoughts could arise.

Also I ask myself now whether my actions take me to light or to darkness. This shows me that when suddenly asked by someone if I'd like to go somewhere while I'm in the middle of doing something, I feel a cut-off, pressurized feeling when I interrupt my activity (which means I move into darkness), whereas most of the time I can move to the light if I simply continue doing what I was occupied with. This is new for me, because I'm accustomed to accepting someone's invitation in order not to be alone and because when I was depressed I used to think that what I was doing was never as good as what the other did.

I find it challenging in my life to make myself a research subject and to experiment with myself; to try things out - to feel what's going on in my body and with my energy when I say something encouraging to myself and what happens when I bring myself down.

Moving to the light doesn't mean that you suppress your pain or feelings like sadness and anger. Experiencing these feelings can also be an expression of purity and sincerity and in this way also an expression of light.

In the brain all nerve cells that have to do with positive experiences are connected with each other. The nerve cells which have to do with negative experiences are also connected with each other. So if you start thinking in a negative way, then all the nerve cells which are associated with that negativity are activated and your thought pattern becomes more and more gloomy. However, if you have the smallest positive thought, you have entered your positive brain.

When depressed, the negative nerve network is activated and it seems as if nothing in your life is right anymore; like you have done everything wrong; like you have only ever experienced negative things in your life. When you are happy, in contrast, the positive network is activated and your whole perspective on that same life changes. Then you feel rich, you feel how blessed you are with all your fulfilling experiences and you consider the depression you have had as a learning period, a necessary passage to something new. So the same events can be experienced in a totally different way, depending on your point of view. There is no absolute truth; our perception is part of it.

The exercise: 'Saying Yes to myself in this moment'

I do the exercise 'saying yes to myself in this moment ' for the first time in Meera Hashimoto's Art Therapy Training. Svagito Liebermeister has described this exercise in his book: *The Zen Way of Counseling*.

It is an exercise to connect with your *being* rather than functioning from your mind (your head). When you say 'yes' to this moment, your minds tends to interfere with everything, because it is the habit of the mind always to want something else, to long for a better future or to compare this moment with the past.

The exercise is this:
First you make sure that you cannot be disturbed and set an alarm clock for fifteen minutes.

Then you start to move, walk around and let your body do whatever it wants. Now you say out loud: 'if I say 'yes' to myself at the moment, I am ...' and then you complete the sentence by describing whatever you find yourself doing in the present moment. For example you may say: 'If I say 'yes' to myself right now, I am wiggling my toes and I am moving my fingers'. Or:' If I say 'yes' to myself right now, I'm yawning'.

Every sentence begins with 'if I say yes to myself ' and is completed by whatever you're doing. It may feel like shrugging your shoulders, laughing, frowning, dancing, rolling around on the floor. Each action should be spontaneous, without calculation or prior intention.

After fifteen minutes you stop, close your eyes and observe your inner state of being.

When I do this exercise, I feel that my mood changes by saying 'yes' in this way. I feel lighter and more carefree because for a few minutes I have not been occupied with worries about the past and the future.

A similar exercise lets you feel the difference between saying 'yes' and saying 'no' to yourself. You can do this exercise when you go for a walk or when are walking around in the city.

During the first five minutes you pronounce again and again the sentence: 'when I say 'no' to myself then….' and you complete that sense with what is there in that moment. For example: 'If I say 'no' to myself I walk with my head down. If I say no to myself I feel irritated with other people. If I say no to myself I don't look around me. If I say no to myself I stamp on the ground.'

After that, for five minutes you repeat the sentence: 'If I say 'yes' to myself then…' and again you complete the sentence with what is happening with you in that moment. For example: 'If I say yes to myself I look around. If I say yes to myself I walk upright and energetically. If I say yes to myself I see colours around me. If I say yes to myself I look at people'.

Notice in yourself if there is a difference between what happens in you when you pronounce the sentence 'If I say 'no' to myself' and the sentence 'If I say 'yes' to myself'.

What I notice when I do this exercise is that when I say 'no' to myself, I seclude myself from everything and everyone and condemn myself and the world around me: I am angry, my fists are clenched, I don't see any colours and I walk bent, with my eyes to the ground.

If I say 'yes' to myself I walk around with my head up, I see colours, have contact with the people around me, feel energetic and look into the world with a positive attitude.

---
*When I say 'yes' to myself I feel energetic
and look into the world with a positive attitude*

Now you can start observing in your own life when you have a 'yes' and when you live from a 'no'. It is important not to say about yourself that you have a 'no' against life, because if you make it so general you don't look accurately at each single moment any more. Even in a depression, little moments can often be found in which you have a 'yes'. From the moment you are aware of your yes-attitude and your no-attitude, you have a choice which attitude you want to choose.

Saying 'no' can be easier. It gives you an identity, a way to define yourself. When you drop your 'no', you thereby also have to drop your ego and open up to the unknown.

Saying 'no' is not always wrong. Sometimes we have to say 'no' to the other if this person asks something from us that we don't want to give, and we have to be able to say 'no' to indicate our boundaries. At such a moment saying 'no' to the other is saying 'yes' to ourselves.

Why is is there so much darkness?

In her book *Dark Night of the Soul* Pamela Kribbe answers the question of why so many people on earth are processing darkness at this time:

"Because you are making a leap forward. It's really a leap in the evolution of consciousness of humanity. That jump cannot be made without reaching out to the darkest places in your consciousness that are filled with fear, distrust or a very deep sadness about all you have been through on earth. Don't be afraid of this, welcome that darkness. When you say yes, it keeps flowing, that is the art. Also when you feel: here I really can't say yes to this, remember that there is still something inside of you that says *yes* anyhow. That will save you and bring you ahead. Trust life.

"By saying yes to the dark and unknown in yourself you will come in contact with the freedom and relaxation associated with self-acceptance."

Processing of darkness has to do with the evolution of human consciousness

---

Osho says about his life:

"In my whole life looking backwards I find that if you are just a little alert everything turns into a blessing. I don't remember anything in my whole life which turned out to be a curse. All nights have proved to be beginnings of a lighter day."*

Saying yes to yourself also means: not comparing yourself with others. Because comparing takes you away from yourself and from the way you have to go. That's what the next chapter is about.

---

* Osho - *From Misery to Enlightenment #1*

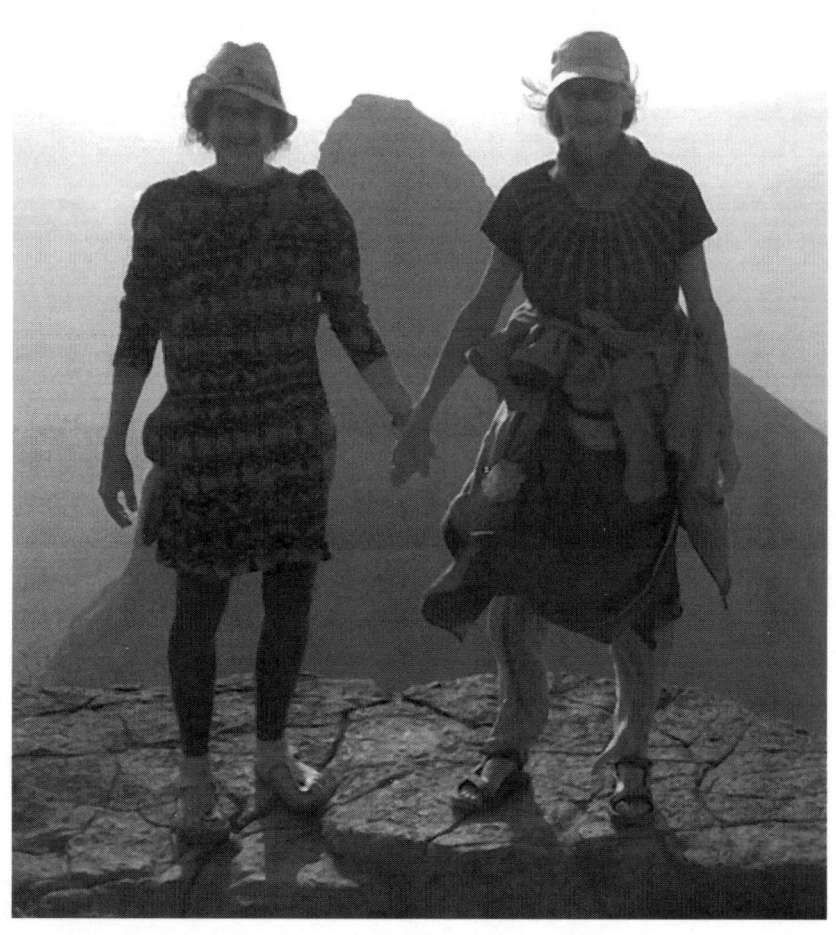

10 STOPPING COMPARING YOURSELF WITH OTHERS BRINGS YOU BACK TO YOURSELF

Envy is wanting something without being willing to pay the price. Instead of working with the envy I prefer to lead the person to a decision point, where he or she may choose to pay the full price for reward and success.*

Bert Hellinger

In my depression I continuously compare myself with others. In every encounter the first thing I do is look to see if the other person's eyes are shining, something I miss in myself. Then I try to live just like that radiant person in order to tap into my happiness through another.

Thus I realise on a sunny morning in Spring - having just got back from India two months previously, where I had been painting with Meera Hashimoto - that Meera is painting cherry blossoms now in Japan with a whole group of peo-

---

* Bert Hellinger - *Acknowledging What Is*

ple, many of whom I know from Pune. I imagine in detail how they will be sitting there now under the abundant, pink blossoms in the bright green Spring grass, each with a piece of plastic to sit on, with a large sheet of paper - handmade in India - and many colours of acrylic paint and ink graded around them. Meera will be speaking to them, inspired by the beauty of Nature, and then be totally absorbed in her own painting. In between, they will be dancing under the blossom trees. That they will experience all this beauty while I don't take part in it is almost unbearable for my gloomy soul.

I decide to make an effort to participate in this too, and fold out my white table on the balcony. On top of it I put a sheet of hand-made blank paper that I have brought from India and bring out my pots of acrylic paint. Then I fill a can with water and put out five different sized brushes. After sitting on my folding chair my eyes connect with my downstairs neighbour's pink blossom tree, which bears thousands of flowers. 'You can only paint what you love', I hear Meera say. So I try to become one with the tree. Then I mix the red and white paint and start. I paint almost without looking at the paper, my eyes focused on the tree; painting as much as possible from my heart. All of a sudden there is a blackbird in the next tree. I want to capture this blackbird in my blossom tree. Firmly I take the black paint and create a cursory sketch of the bird, just as it flies up and comes down in a lateral position. Well, then I will paint that aspect too. Now there are two blackbirds in my tree. I see myself and my unborn twin sister in it. Right now I'm really satisfied.

Then I am overwhelmed by homesickness; for Meera and for the painting process with her. This takes me all of a sudden far away from my painting; far away from my blossom tree. My mind is in Japan again. I imagine them eating together there and reflect that I myself can never be as nice as any of them. My satisfaction is gone and the passion which my brush still had in painting the blackbird has flown off. It feels like being cross-eyed; my one eye sees the blossom tree before my balcony, while my other eye is focused on Japan. In my chest it feels like a wrung-out mop, called: comparison.

*By comparing myself with others
my creativity disappears*

Turning towards myself is not attractive because then I enter the dry, grey desert which is there. I hope for a 'shortcut' to somebody else's happiness.

I was once told that even if I had what belonged to the other, it probably wouldn't make me happy because it's not my own. Even though I presume that this person is right I still can't imagine being happy with anything which is mine. The gold of the other glitters so much.

I think that comparing myself to others started when my sister was born, when I was one year old. Up until that time, I had been the only child and had felt that part of my mother's attention was always somewhere else, probably with her experiences in the concentration camp. I did my best to be seen. When another baby came I interpreted it as meaning I wasn't good enough for my parents. When all the attention went to my sister, I thought that she must definitely have something which made her better than who I was.

The more I compare myself with others, the further I drift away from my own core. And yet I keep doing it. It is a kind of addiction, one which I almost cannot overcome any more. It gives me a pseudo-life; it looks like I'm living the life of the person with whom I compare, just like watching a movie in which I identify with the main character. When the movie is over, I tumble down with a bang, back into my own reality. Maybe having compared myself so long with others I have reached finally a point where I can see how destructive comparison is, consuming and undermining me inside, and that anything is better than this. At last from this deep realisation I begin to know that the only place from where I can start to change is this very one where I am right now: this very moment. Even if this is the darkest place in the world it is always better to be here than comparing myself to someone else's light place. As soon as I transfer myself into someone else's place - literally or in my mind - I let go of the rope that connects me with myself, and I become a piece of driftwood that floats alongside the person to whom I am comparing myself in that moment.

*As soon as I start comparing with another,
I lose the connection with myself*

It is a tough exercise to change over every time I catch myself thinking 'I wish I had what the other has', to checking with myself 'where am I now' and 'how do I feel inside'.

I regularly recall the encounter I had with a boy whom I met - on my trip to India - at the airport in a small coffee shop. I told him about the meditation centre I was going to. The boy looked at me seriously and said, 'I have travelled a lot, but I learned most at the most boring places, with the most boring people, in the most boring circumstances'.

This sentence has always remained with me because I had already assumed that there would come a time when I would have to stay between the - in my eyes - dull buildings of the Netherlands in order just to pay attention to myself and to enter consciously into myself.

Now I have found the connection with myself, I see how I can only enjoy, experience satisfaction and feel fulfilment in something which truly belongs to me; by being connected with myself. It is better even to feel sad or agitated than to compare myself with someone else.

---

*Even when I feel very sad or restless,
it is better than comparing myself with someone else*

Moreover, the image I had of someone else during my depression was mostly not correct. Many people often put a smile on their face to hide their pain, just like me. And the photos on Facebook are only a snapshot of an occasion when someone feels good at that moment, while sometimes this person is not happy the rest of the time. I see now how much I have projected onto others what I was missing in myself.

High Sensitivity: scanning the feelings of the other

Fons Delnooz and Patricia Martinot describe in their *Handbook of Energetic Protection* how when you have felt emotionally unsafe as a child, you have started to develop very sensitive tentacles to scan your environment. As a result, the energy field around you - your aura - has become too big. Energetically you no longer live inside your body but outside, in your aura. You are then very capable of scanning the feelings of others and you are also very strongly influenced by those feelings of other people. It can feel very unsafe to return to yourself in your body because you have much less sense of what is happening around you then.

Where as a highly sensitive child I had the tendency to be continuously occupied with scanning the feelings of others, in my depressions this took unhealthy forms. I started considering the feelings of others as more important than my own feelings, because in myself I encountered nothing but greyness and drabness. It became a welcome distraction to think about the weal and woe of the other and to remain concentrated on that.

---

*I started considering the feelings of others
as more important than my own feelings*

In the *Handbook of Energetic Protection* Fons Delnooz and Patricia Martinot provide exercises that can bring you back to yourself. I often use the one of imaging a parachute, in which by pulling on its strings I bring myself back to myself. I restore the energy to my own centre this way, as soon as I notice that it's transferred completely to someone else.

In the beginning it felt very selfish and also quite lonely; I was no longer intertwined with others. But gradually it has started to feel like a new acquired freedom: I can now choose to stay with myself. As a result, I have much more energy, which I can use for myself and, if I choose, also to make contact with another person, without losing myself in him or her.

In the process of coming out of my depression I have experienced that the body is the foundation of making connection with myself and with the other. The body is honest and has an incredible wisdom. This is the subject of the next part of this book.

Part 3

Healing from the Body

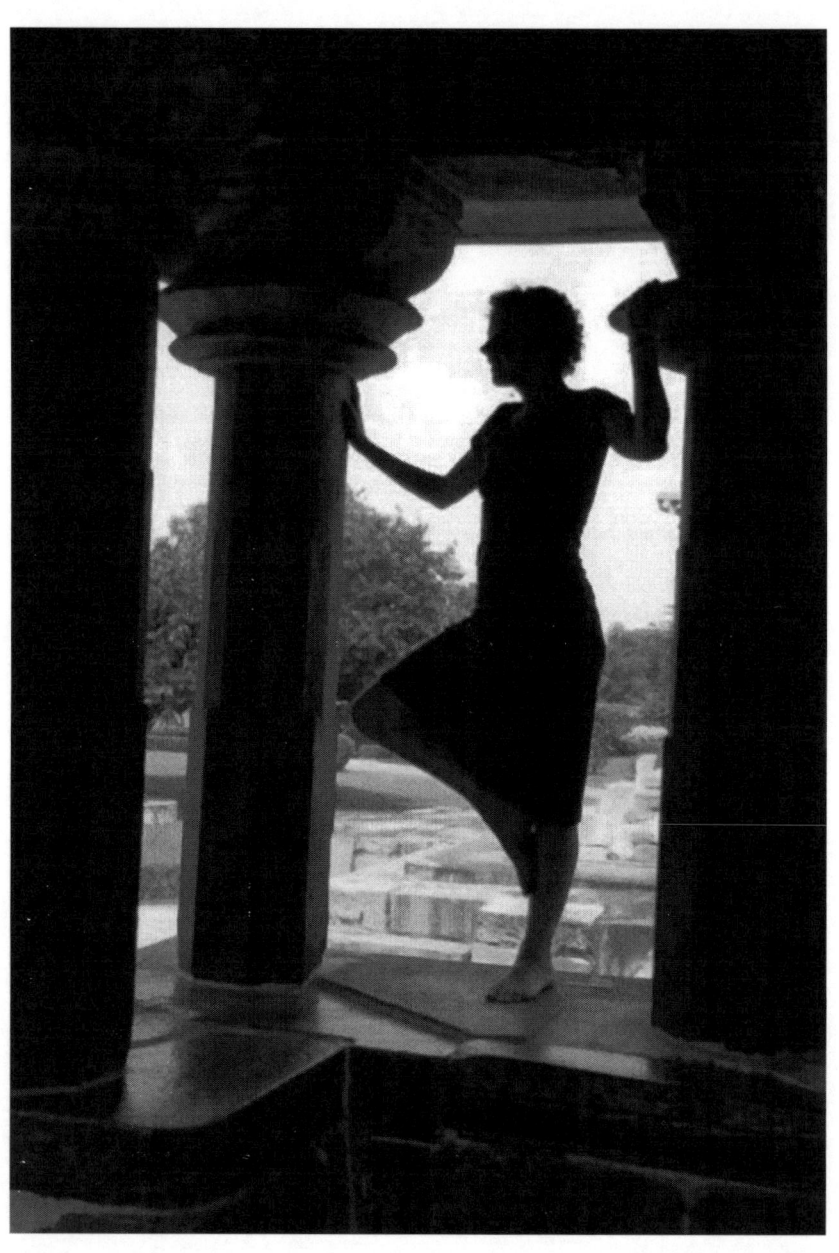

11 YOUR BODY IS THE BASIS OF GOOD THERAPY

Body and Emotions are connected

Love is therapy, and there is no other therapy in the world except love. It is always love that heals, because love makes you whole, love makes you feel welcome in the world, love makes you a part of existence. It destroys alienation. Then you are no more an outsider here, but utterly needed. Love makes you feel needed, and to be needed is the greatest need. Nothing else can fulfill that great need. Unless you feel that you are contributing something to existence, unless you feel that without you the existence would be a little less, that you would be missed, that you are irreplaceable, you will not feel healthy and whole.*

Osho

When depressed, I use my mind to try to find the solution to get out of it.

I dive deep into my past to see if I can find a clue there for my unhappiness. That does me no good; more and more unfortunate episodes from my life reveal themselves. The whole nerve network involved in the storage of sad events is activated. I regret everything from my past and criticise the choices

---

* Osho - *The Secret of Secrets # 18*

I have made. The more I dive into the past, the more hopeless my situation seems to be.

Besides that I try to plan a bright future, not realising that a picture of the future is just an extension of something that you already know. From my gloomy state of being my future expectations can't therefore be anything other than worrying. I can't imagine the future very different from what I can conceive of right now.

I find it scary to let go of my thoughts about the past and the future. They seem to be my only hold. And the more strongly I become occupied with past and future, the narrower the straitjacket is that I pull around me. My perception through the senses is strongly coloured by my dark thoughts. I interpret everything I see around me negatively; dull grey buildings, deathly dull streets, fast moving, unattainable people. The dullness that I see around me is a reflection of what I experience in myself: deadness; because I have lost the connection with myself and with everything around me.

The dullness that I see around me is a reflection of what I experience in myself

---

In depression the emotions are suppressed

Pamela Kribbe describes in her book *Dark Night of the Soul* how you start closing yourself off out of self-protection when emotions become too overwhelming. Out of self-protection you start resisting what's coming into your life and create a 'no' to life. You hide your feelings, hoping to feel better again. Often however the opposite happens, because emotions are an essential part of life. They tell you how you feel, how you experience certain situations and what your expectations are. You are happy, disappointed, angry, scared, sad; your emotions make you feel you are living.

Without emotions you are basically dead and cut off from everything and everyone around you. This is so unbearable that you can consider putting an end to your life. The longer you turn off your emotions, the more difficult it becomes even to feel them. But life has a driving force which ensures that you cannot remain constantly in the same state of consciousness. Just at the moment that you have reached the lowest point, from your soul a counterforce comes into effect. You create happenings in your life then, which ensure that a passage, a change occurs.

Pamela has experienced this from her own night of the soul and sees it happening to the people she guides in their spiritual growth and awareness.

The emotional centre in the brain is located in the limbic system. In our evolution, that is one of the oldest areas in our brain. It is responsible for our psychological well-being and controls a large part of the physiology of our body as well: heart function, blood pressure, hormones, digestion and the immune system.

The limbic system is barely in contact with our neocortex (which in evolutionary terms is seen as the newest part of our brain, the part that ensures we can reason, argue, plan, speak, understand and control our impulses), but the limbic system is in direct contact with our body, through the involuntary nervous system.

That's why therapy that only works via thinking and language has little effect. It is necessary to involve the body and even to take the body as a starting point.

Therapy that only works via thinking has little effect;
it is necessary to involve the body

The value of the emotional brain

In his book *Healing without Freud or Prozac* psychiatrist Dr. David Servan-Schreiber describes how depression is caused by an imbalance in the emotional brain. We are happy when the emotional brain and our neocortex work together; thereby the emotional brain gives us direction in what we want with our lives, while our cognitive brain helps to put this into effect. When you use the cognitive brain too much (too much thinking and analyzing), you can't hear the signals that the emotional brain sends you any longer. Your real choices come from your emotional brain. When you do not have access to this brain anymore, you can no longer make choices and you are rudderless.

When we do not have access to our emotions
we can no longer make choices

Dr. Servan-Schreiber describes in the above mentioned book* that the cause of the poor functioning of the emotional brain usually comes from painful experiences in the past. These are stored in the nervous system although they are already over. As a result, in your present situation you still react as if you were in that previous painful situation. With the help of psychotherapy you can re-programme the emotional brain

---

* Dr Servan Schreiber - *Healing without Freud or Prozac*

again. Since this brain is especially connected with the body, it enables you to work through the body more effectively than through methods that appeal to thinking.

So this is immediately the major disadvantage of antidepressants: they flatten the emotions and disturb the balance of the body, thus closing-off the main access points for psychotherapy.

Already in 1890 Professor William James, father of American psychology, wrote that emotion is first and foremost a condition of the body and only as a secondary condition is sensed in the brain.

The goal of therapy is to help you see the unnatural in yourself

Our upbringing has taught us rules to enable us to survive in our society. As a result our neocortex is programmed in such a way that we have gradually moved away from our true self and have become increasingly unnatural.

Somebody asks Osho: Is the purpose of the therapy groups to bring the participants to their natural self?

Osho answers:

"The purpose of the therapy groups is not to bring the participants to their natural self - not at all. The purpose of the therapy groups is to bring you to the point where you can see your unnaturalness.

"The natural can exist without your co-operation, but the unnatural cannot exist. The unnatural needs constant support, it needs constant care, it needs constant control. Once you have seen that: 'this is unnatural', your grip on it becomes loose. Your fist opens of its own accord.

"The group is not a device to open your fist. It is just to help you see that what you are doing is unnatural. In that very seeing, the transformation.

"The purpose of the therapy groups is just to make the participants aware of the unnatural self. And then the natural self comes of its own accord. Nobody can bring it - when the unnatural disappears, the natural is found.

"The natural has always been there, hidden under the rubbish. Unnatural gone, you are natural. You don't become natural; you have always been natural. How can one become natural? All becoming will lead you into unnaturalness.

"Nobody can make you natural - God has already done that.*

When the unnatural disappears the natural emerges

Choose a therapist who works from Love

When you choose therapy, it is important to find a good therapist. Only when the therapist acts from love, respect and awareness and himself lives in coherence with what he extols, along with there being a click between you and the therapist, can therapy be effective.

Love is healing. And the emotional brain - which we especially address in therapy - does not listen to words but to the way in which something is said, to the sound of the voice; the hardness, the pitch, the energy with which the words are expressed and the haste or calmness with which they are spoken. It looks at the eyes of the therapist: are these loving or tense and impatient?

---

* Osho - *Take it Easy #12*

A good therapist is not out to change you but creates a climate in which you yourself make your own discoveries.

A good therapist is not out to change you but creates a climate in which you yourself make your discoveries

---

Osho: "There is only one way of loving people: love them as they are. And this is the beauty: that when you love them as they are, they change. Not according to you - they change according to *their* reality. When you love them, they are transformed - not converted, transformed. They become new, they attain newer heights of being. But that happens in their being, and it happens according to their nature."*

Pamela Kribbe writes in her book *Dark Night of the Soul*: "If someone sees your divine core and makes contact with your soul at a moment when you cannot temporarily do this yourself, that feels to you as if you were called by your real name. Nothing is so empowering and healing as to be called by your real name. It means that someone sees you as you are, in your true nature: radiant, powerful and sincere."

In the Art Therapy Training with Meera Hashimoto I experienced how healing it was to be called by my real name. Meera's love and respect meant I could begin to make the changes that were necessary for me.

Nothing is as healing as being seen by someone as you are, in your true nature: radiant, powerful and sincere

---

* Osho - *Come Follow to You, Vol 2 #6*

Body-oriented Therapy forms

Below I describe a number of body-oriented therapy forms, which I can recommend.

These are: Primal Rebirth® Therapy, Gestalt Therapy, Bio Energetics, Emotional Bodywork, Craniosacral Therapy, Rebalancing, Haptotherapy and Acupuncture. In addition, I can recommend the technique of Heart Coherence and Singing.

On the cognitive level I have, as I have described, benefited from Schema Therapy to help me see the patterns in which I was stuck.

Here is a brief description of these various forms of therapy.

Primal Rebirth® therapy

Primal Rebirth® therapy is a profound form of therapy. It is a spiritual growth therapy developed by Omkar Dingjan and Divyam Kranenburg, founders of the Aumm Institute. The therapy is in fact an investigation that gives you the opportunity to get to know your inner child and to become aware of the fact that your past still plays an important role in your life; your early childhood is the origin of most of the problems you have.

By experiencing and feeling the child in yourself, asking it questions, accepting and starting to love it, you can recognize any beliefs and survival mechanisms that limit you and then let go of them. From an attitude of acceptance, the child within you can become detached from the past and return to its original essence hand in hand with the adult in yourself, who is strengthened by this therapy.

To achieve this, a number of techniques are used, through which you come into contact with yourself physically, emotionally and spiritually. Meditation is an important part of this work.*

In your early childhood lies the origin of most of the problems you have

---

Gestalt Therapy

Gestalt is the German word for 'whole'. Gestalt therapy works with the way you experience yourself as a whole.

The goal of the therapy is to remove the blockages that prevent your growth, in order that further growth becomes possible again and your mental problems reduce.

Bio Energetics

Bioenergetics is based on the unity of body and mind. Painful experiences in your life are stored in the body in the form of muscular tensions. Bio-energetic therapy is aimed at releasing those tensions by means of physical exercises and re-initiating the balance and energy flow in your body again.

Painful experiences in your life are stored in the body in the form of muscular tensions

---

* Aumm instituut [Aumm institute] - www.aumm.nl

Emotional Bodywork

In emotional body work you get back in touch with your body and the tensions which are stored in it through the physical, using breathing techniques, voice work and exercises involving discharge, effort and relaxation. You become aware of the signals that your body gives you and of the emotions that go with them. You learn to accept and appreciate your emotions. All kinds of feelings, which were often suppressed before, can be released - such as anger, fear and frustration. By living through those feelings you start feeling more free and vital.

Craniosacral Therapy

In Craniosacral therapy the practitioner connects through gentle touch with the rhythm of the craniosacral system, which surrounds the central nervous system. Many tensions are created by the imbalance of our nervous system. With craniosacral therapy these tensions can be dissolved, creating more space, balance and relaxation.

Rebalancing

Rebalancing is a body-oriented therapy that gives you more insight into yourself. You learn to relax the cramping your body and mind have become accustomed to in the course of your life. This relaxation gives a sense of well-being and helps you to move from thinking to conscious feeling, and from conscious feeling to your *being*. By being actively present in the body every physical experience can become an opening to your inner world and to new insights into yourself.

Rebalancing was originally created in the Osho Meditation Centre from the merging of Western forms of bodywork with the Eastern meditative approach of Osho.

Haptotherapy

The purpose of Haptotherapy is to get in touch with and gain trust in your own feelings again. Haptotherapy guides you through your psychological symptoms to the point where they can be processed emotionally. You become aware of the information that a touch gives you about your emotional life, and of the way in which you live. This awareness can create a sense of security, balance and self-confidence.

Acupuncture

An acupuncture treatment brings the involuntary nervous system into balance; it can balance the calming parasympathetic nervous system with the activating sympathetic nervous system. When the involuntary nervous system is in balance, the emotional brain (that is directly connected with this nervous system) comes into balance too.

Heart Coherence

A healthy heart does not always beat at the same speed. The rhythm varies with breathing. When you are in a state of well-being, this variance (the heart coherence) forms a regular pattern; then there is high heart coherence. When you are depressed, tense or anxious, a chaotic pattern in the variation of the heart rhythm develops; the heart coherence is low then.

With high heart coherence your brain, heart, nervous system and hormone system work optimally together. You feel energetic and healthy and you can think clearly.

In the book *Healing without Freud or Prozac* Dr. David Servan-Schreiber describes how the heart and the emotional brain are directly connected to each other by tens of thousands of nerve cells and hormones, causing a direct interaction between the emotional brain and the heart. By learning to control your heart coherence you can directly bring your emotional brain into harmony.

The heart and the emotional brain are directly connected to each other

---

The exercise I practise myself to increase heart coherence is the following:

You breathe in for a count of four, imagining that your breath enters through the heart area. Then you breathe out for six counts, imagining that your breath leaves through the abdominal area. You only have to do the exercise for a few minutes.

There are apps that can be downloaded for the guidance of the breath.

By increasing heart coherence, balance is created in the involuntary nervous system and this allows you to respond calmly to anything that happens in your daily life.

You will be able to access much more easily your intuition and your emotions. You will have more compassion for yourself and thereby also for others.

Heart coherence is a technique you can apply anywhere whenever you find yourself out of balance. The technique creates a better connection with your inner self.

Self-activation method for overcoming Depression

Psychologist Willem van de Sanden has developed a self-activation therapy outlined in his book *Depressie Actief Overwinnen [Active Overcoming Depression]*.

In the book he describes depression in a clear and comprehensible way and provides a self-help method to get out of depression. You work on connecting better with your body, making contact with others, sleeping better, exercising and relaxation.

About feelings and emotions he writes:

"If you run away from feelings, your feelings stay on top of you. For example, when you can admit to yourself that you are afraid or get tense about certain things, that is the first step in the direction of getting less scared or tense. Feelings and emotions are not good or bad. They are sources of information. Feelings and emotions are also related to how you look at the world and how you deal with it. You can indirectly influence your feelings by changing something in your way of thinking and in what you do.

"When there is a lot of tension, the desire of course will arise to relax. However you are tense for the reason that you want to suppress your feelings. So if you relax then, very unpleasant feelings may be coming up. That is why it is important also to develop a strategy to deal with your problems and difficulties.

"And for this, therapy and meditation are very suitable." *

---

*If you start relaxing,
very unpleasant feelings may be coming up.
For this, therapy and meditation are very suitable*

Singing

The throat chakra (the energy centre at the level of the throat) is blocked in a lot of people. That's because from a very early age our voice is frequently silenced: 'say this, don't say that, don't sing out of tune, don't shout so loud' and so on. Because of this we have already started to tighten our throat muscles, so that we will not accidentally utter something wrong.

The throat chakra is the centre of expression, of creativity. In depression this centre is often suppressed.

Singing, in the shower for example, can help to open this again. In singing, you can express your feelings. It doesn't matter whether you can keep the right pitch or not. What is important is that there is discharge, that space is created and that you can give expression to yourself.

I have noticed that when I am worrying, my worries disappear like snow before the sun when I start singing in the shower. Singing is in any case associated with cheerfulness.

---

* Willem van de Sanden - *Depressie Actief Overwinnen [Active Overcoming Depression]*

I sometimes even love to sing solemn songs in a minor key. The singing always gives me a feeling of flow - my head gets empty and I start breathing more deeply.

You can also use movement to start your energy flow. This is the subject of the next chapter.

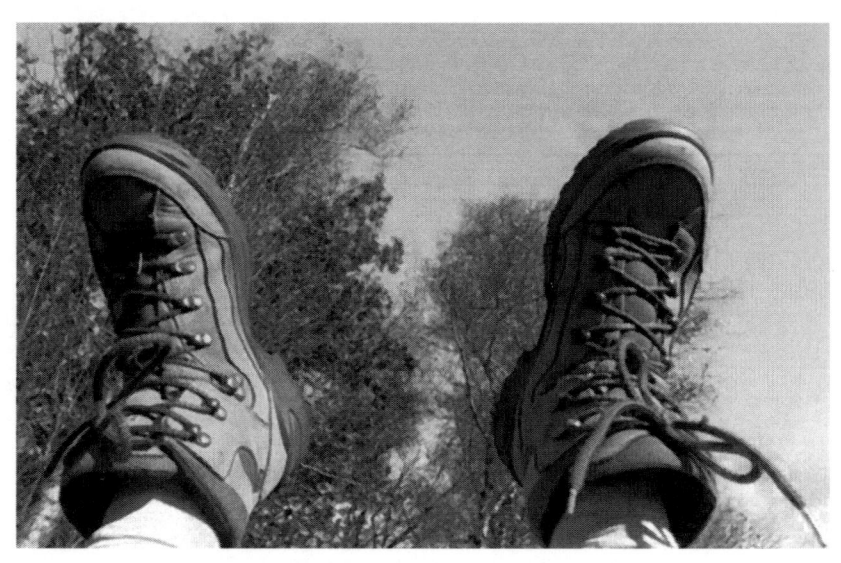

12 PHYSICAL EXERCISE WITH AWARENESS

"If you can run then there is no need for any other meditation - it is enough. Any action in which you can be total becomes meditation, and running is so beautiful that you can be totally lost in it. And you are in contact with all the elements - the sun, the air, the earth, the sky; you are in contact with existence.
When you are running totally, thinking stops.
And in those moments of non-thinking, your existence is pure, you simply are, you don't know who. You don't know who you are. All is forgotten, you are unburdened of the head; you are again an animal. In that moment - when you are again an animal - there is a possibility to contact godliness. Before we can rise high and reach the ultimate we will have to become authentic, as authentic as animals. Through running that authenticity happens."*

Osho

When I am depressed, there are two opposing currents going on in me: on the one hand I feel I have no energy and from deep inside resist every shift of my muscles. On the other hand everything in me wants to move, in a restlessness that

---

* Osho - *This Is It* #12

drives me outside and forces me to walk in endless rounds in the neighbourhood in which I live. It is the restlessness of wanting to do something in the world that is meaningful and in which my energy can flow, without being able to find an outlet for that.

When a psychotherapist proposes to me - during my stay in the psychiatric unit of the hospital - to start running every morning, at first everything in me resists this idea. I am not in touch with my body and cannot imagine that something physical will take me out of my depression. Nevertheless, I want to try it out and start having a good run in the morning before the therapy begins. To my surprise I notice that while running, my energy comes back; I breathe the fresh air, feel my heart beating, smell the trees and plants and my thoughts disappear into the background.

I manage to keep doing it for a week. Then I lack the discipline to continue, despite the good effect it had. It seems that at least three months are needed before a good habit really becomes so much a part of you that you start longing for it every day.

While I am running my energy comes back

Later the Osho Dynamic Meditation, which I return to later in this book, becomes my form of physical activity.

Physical activity has a beneficial effect on depression

Exercise, even when only a small amount of physical activity, has a beneficial effect on depression. When you are active for twenty minutes or more, the depressive thoughts stop during the exercise and after a while there are automatically positive thoughts. A creative thinking process often starts happening as well. It's good not to move in an unconscious way (such as watching television while exercising at the gym) but to be aware of your body while moving. For example, you can observe your breathing or what happens to your feet when they hit the ground. In this way you remain in the moment, in which usually no problem can be found.

The brain releases endorphins and norepinephrine when the body is active, substances that give a feeling of happiness. Heart coherence, which I mentioned in the previous chapter, is also promoted, and the nervous system becomes balanced.

Sustained movement for at least twenty minutes three times a week can establish these positive effects. It is important that you do not force yourself when doing this, but pay close attention to the limit of your abilities. It is from this point your growth starts, your energy starts flowing.

Physical exercise makes your body producing happiness hormones

---

Physical Exercise is needed to be able to relax

Osho: "If a person is to relax, he will have to pass through a state of absolute tension; it is only then that the passage to relaxation becomes possible. If a man works throughout the day, he can sleep well in the night. The harder he works, the deeper he sleeps. The truth is that relaxation follows tension as night follows day, as the valley follows the peak. The higher the peak, the deeper the valley.

"That is how, when your tension grows, at the same time you are gathering energy to relax and rest. The higher the summit of tension, the deeper the valley of rest. That is the reason I ask you to bring all your energy into it, to exert your best, to stake your all and not to withhold yourself even a little bit. That is how you will reach the height of tension and then descend into the bottomless pit of relaxation and rest. And it is in that moment of absolute rest that meditation happens."*

---

*If somebody wants to relax
he first has to pass through a state of absolute tension*

Yoga, Tai Chi and Qi Gong

Yoga, Tai Chi and Qi Gong are forms of conscious exercise which in depression can help to restore the connection with the body and to promote emotional well-being.

Yoga

Shannon Paige is a yoga teacher. She came into contact with yoga when she got cancer. While doing the yoga exercises she began to feel that moving the body can change the spirit and can be healing for both mental and emotional well-being. In a TED talk she says: "Placing your foot behind your head and other difficult yoga postures do not repair your life. Yoga heals no depression. But being-in-your-body can do that. An

---

* Osho - *In Search of the Miraculous #6*

important role in this is the body-mind-breathing connection that is created by conscious exercise, such as Yoga, Tai Chi and Qi Gong." *

Being-in-your-body consciously, can heal depression

Tai Chi, Qi Gong

'Qi' is life force. Tai Chi and Qi Gong are harmonious body movements carried out in a state of concentrated rest. A flow arises in your body when you move in this subtle way, a feeling of liveliness in which at the same time you also experience peace.

Tai Chi and Qi Gong have helped me to feel my body as a complete whole again and to let my life energy flow from my feet to my crown. Since my high school years I have been standing and walking with my head bent forward and my shoulders raised. In Qi Gong classes I feel that everything in my body starts to flow when I stand straight with my shoulders in a neutral position, and this makes me want to compose the correct posture from inside myself.

Through Qi Gong space is created in my body: between the joints, between the muscles and also between the vertebrae, so that all the nerves get more space. The whole body is energised by the good flow of energy. By training the consciousness a connection is created with all organs, muscles and bones.

I also come across blockages (pain points), around which I now carefully move instead of fighting with them. Gradually these blockages resolve, creating a sense of joy, energy and freedom.

---

* YouTube: TEDxBoulder - Shannon Paige - *Mindfulness and Healing*

Through Qi Gong I adopt the right posture from inside, which releases my energy to flow
---

Of course there are many other ways of moving than running, yoga, tai chi or qi gong.

It is important that you choose the way of moving that suits you best; then you have the most fun and it takes no effort to keep it going. A positive spiral starts happening this way: the more you move, the more you feel like moving.

Just as exercise causes the release of substances that give you a feeling of happiness, so can the right food do this. The next chapter is about food.

13 FOOD AND DEPRESSION

The right food makes the eyes shine and lets the heart speak. *

Fons Delnooz & Patricia Martinot

While I am depressed I don't want to think about healthy eating and drinking. I do not value myself enough to delve into this subject and at the time I am convinced that my depression has nothing to do with it.

In my depression I deny the influence of nutrition on my body and on my mood

---

* Fons Delnooz & Patricia Martinot - *Voeding en Spiritualiteit [Diet and Spirituality]*

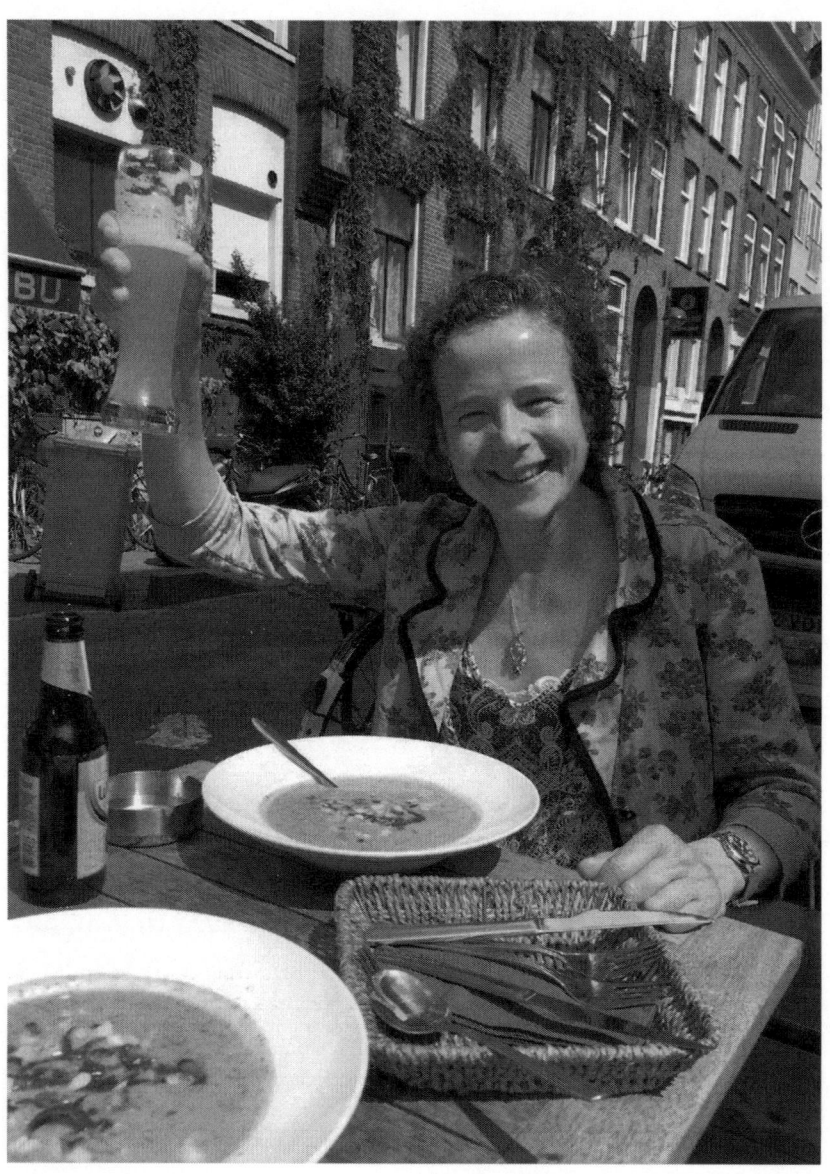

On a dark winter morning, when it's raining cats and dogs and when I am more gloomy than ever, I cycle to the railway station and at the snack bar there order a portion of greasy chips with a thick blob of mayonnaise. I start eating it on the floor at the station's exit, where the drenched boots of the travellers pass by, splattering mud. This setting exactly fits the feeling I have. It is also a revolt against everyone who gives me advice on healthy eating.

I want to resolve my depression only through consciousness. By the time I come out of my final depression, I have started to feel that my body is an important source of happiness and that a good diet makes my body lively and resilient. I notice then how much the food I eat influences my mood and consciousness. My arrogance towards my physical self is over.

The right food brings you into your power

In their book *Voeding en Spiritualiteit [Food and Spirituality]* Fons Delnooz and Patricia Martinot describe the importance of carefully selecting food which is also well grown and well processed (organic or biodynamic food) to create balance in your body and for the flow of your life energy. The energy flow released by consuming this food, opens you for who you essentially are. By observing very carefully what effect on you the food you take has, you gradually start feeling which food you need. That is quite different to choosing what is tasty or what fills your stomach.

"If man continuously eats and drinks what he really needs, he continually knows who he is and a force arises in him. This force we call 'the bearing middle'. This bearing middle is a life guide. It continually shows man if he is still on the right track. This man knows: I am power, I am love, I am light."*

If man continuously eats and drinks what he really needs, he continually knows who he is and a force arises in him

---

In their book Delnooz and Martinot describe how difficult it is when you are out of balance to be able to select food that suits you and which will bring you back into that equilibrium.

In the West - accustomed as we are to the many stimuli around us – we have also become accustomed to tantalizing food; food with a lot of sugars as well as coffee. We often think only of what fills up our stomach and of eating something tasty, but not of what can give us energy and make us vital. The vegetables in the supermarket are often sprayed with poison and grown in greenhouses without light or real soil, resulting in the vegetables lacking life force. Because of this the products of the current food industry are often empty, without any nutritional value and with many sugars added.

When you eat empty food you yourself feel empty also: you are what you eat. From that void you tend to do other things which correspond with this void, such as surfing channels on television, playing computer games, eating whole bags of crisps or - just like me - sitting on the floor at the station's exit with greasy chips.

---

* Fons Delnooz and Patricia Martinot - *Voeding en Spiritualiteit [Food and Spirituality]*

Fons Delnooz and Patricia Martinot call the negative spiral in which you then end up the 'circle of imbalance'. It requires a lot of awareness and discipline to break that circle. If you have eaten empty and tantalizing food for a long time, it is very difficult to understand the signals from your body and to feel which food is good for you.

When you have managed to make yourself choose healthy food (such as high-quality fresh vegetables, fresh fruit, water, herbal tea), you usually end up in a void at first, where everything seems to have lost its lustre. This is because the adrenaline in your body caused by the tempting food is not present anymore. When your determination allows you to endure this, you gradually come to a 'circle of balance'; your nervous system comes to rest, you can concentrate better, you are more in touch with your natural rhythm of waking and sleeping and you can open yourself to love, consciousness and the light within yourself. You start seeing and feeling more clearly who you really are.

When your body comes into balance with the right nutrition you can open yourself to values like love, consciousness and the light within yourself

---

The impact that diet has on mental well-being is not sufficiently acknowledged by doctors; in medical training there is still far too little education about this subject. Fortunately, there are doctors who pick up this important issue. They have united in the association 'Doctors and Nutrition'.*

---

* Website of Arts en Voeding [Doctor and Nourishment]: www.voedingonline.nl

Food has a great influence on all the hormones in the body as well as on the production of happiness hormones. A book that illustrates this clearly is *het Energieke Vrouwen Voedingskompas [The Women's Energetic Nutritional Compass]* by Marjolein Dubbers. The book is also suitable for men.

Below I describe the beneficial effect on depression of estrogens, omega-3, yellow root powder, vitamin D, fermented foods, vitamin B, folic acid and saffron, and the importance of avoiding coffee, alcohol and nicotine as much as possible. In addition, I describe how important it is to make sure that the intestines – the largest producer of happiness hormones - are healthy.

The antidepressant effect of estrogens

In and after menopause as well as in the second half of the menstrual cycle, women produce fewer estrogens. As a result, less of the happiness hormone serotonin is created. This can result in depression and anxiety. Marjolein Dubbers describes in her book *'het Energieke Vrouwen Voedingskompas' [The Women's Energetic Nutritional Compass]* how you can supplement this shortage with the right nutrition.

Omega-3 reduces depression symptoms

In his book *Healing without Freud or Prozac* psychiatrist Dr. David Servan-Schreiber points out that research shows that depression symptoms are reduced by half within a few weeks when Omega-3 intake is sufficient.

Omega-3 is built into the wrapping of nerve cells and makes those nerve cells more flexible. It also increases the production of neurotransmitters (substances that provide for the transfer of the stimuli of nerve cells) in the emotional part of the brain and puts you in a good mood and helps you experience more fun.

Since the Second World War our food has started to contain much less Omega-3 and when we do not take extra Omega-3 through our diet, we have by definition a shortage of this important fatty acid. Omega-3 is for example in mackerel, anchovies (in their entirety, not as fillet), sardine, herring, tuna, haddock and trout. Vegetable sources are linseed oil, hemp oil, walnuts, purslane leaves, spinach, seaweed and spirulina.

It is important that Omega-3 and Omega-6 are balanced in our diet. An excess of Omega-6 provokes inflammatory reactions in the body and inflammatory reactions can cause depression.

Depression symptoms are reduced by half within a few weeks when you get enough Omega-3

The intestines produce the neurotransmitters serotonin and dopamine, which provide a feeling of happiness

The intestinal bacteria produce no less than ninety-five percent of the serotonin supply; so the intestines are also called 'the second brain.' Also dopamine is for the most part produced by these bacteria. It is necessary to plan your diet in such a way that the good intestinal bacteria that provide this production, proliferate.

It is also necessary that your diet contains the proteins that are needed to make serotonin and dopamine.

Fermented food (that is food that is converted by bacteria, fungi and yeasts) is the best food to bring about healthy intestinal flora.

Examples of fermented foods are organic yogurt, sauerkraut, kefir, miso, tempeh and some chutneys.

Probiotics can also bring good bacterial flora into your intestines.

The most important thing is that you eat a wide range of fresh foods that have not been processed, because the more variety in what you eat, the more varied the composition of the good bacteria in your intestines is.

A lot of information can be found on the internet. Among other places:
- on the website of Marojolein Dubbers: energiekevrouwenacademie.nl [only in Dutch]
- on the website of osteopathic doctor Dr. Mercola: www.mercola.com

In the following books you will find good information:
- *Het Energieke Vrouwen Voedingskompas [The Women's Energetic Nutritional Compass]* by Marjolein Dubbers
- *Food Pharmacy* by Lina Nerthby Aurell & Mia Clase
- *Voeding en Spiritualiteit [Food and Spirituality]* by Fons Delnooz & Patricia Martinot

---

A healthy intestinal flora provides vitality and a good mood

Depression can be the result of a chronic bowel inflammation

Depression is often the result of a chronic inflammation of the intestinal wall. This inflammation occurs when too many free radicals are formed in the body, which damage the intestinal wall. An excess of free radicals arises, for example, if you follow a wrong diet, have a lot of stress, do not exercise and smoke. The chronic inflammation causes a disturbance in the balance between good and bad bacteria and the bad bacteria start predominating. The production of serotonin and dopamine then decreases and you get a shortage of many other nutrients because they can no longer be properly absorbed by the intestinal wall. All of this affects your mood negatively. The intestines also harbour the largest proportion (seventy to eighty percent) of the body's immune system. For this reason, with a chronic inflammation of the intestinal wall, your resistance against bacteria, viruses, fungi, yeasts, and parasites is very low and you become ill very easily.

You can help your body to defend itself against free radicals by using food that stimulates good intestinal bacteria.

Depression can be the result of a chronic inflammation of the intestines

---

Yellow root powder has an antidepressant effect

Turmeric (yellow root powder) has an antidepressant effect. It causes the release of dopamine and serotonin and protects the nerves.

It must be linked to a supplement (black pepper) because otherwise it is not properly absorbed by the intestines.

Turmeric also prevents inflammation. This is particularly important for people with depression, because intestinal inflammations so often contribute to depression or even underlie it.

Vitamin D makes your mood shine

Almost everyone knows the healing effect of sunlight. Under the influence of sunlight the skin can make vitamin D. Vitamin D has an antidepressant effect. The more you can be in the sun, the better it is for vitamin D production. Fatty fish also contains vitamin D, but it is very difficult to get enough of this vitamin through the diet. The vitamin D requirement increases with age. It is therefore necessary to take Vitamin D supplements for women over fifty and men over seventy years old.

Sugars contribute to depression

It is healthy to eat as few sugars as possible, because they have many harmful effects. As far as depression is concerned, the following is important here:

High blood sugars increase the levels of the hormone insulin in the blood and that causes inflammation in the body. Inflammation in the intestines disrupts the healthy bacteria that produce serotonin and dopamine. The sugars feed the bad bacteria in the intestines, so that the good ones do not have enough space to do their work.

In order to process sugar in the body, auxiliary substances such as the vitamins-B are required. When you eat a lot of sugars, a vitamin B deficiency quickly develops, which can lead to depression.

You can use honey occasionally instead of sugar.

Eating a lot of sugars creates a vitamin B deficiency which can cause depression

---

Vitamin B, folic acid and Saffron have depression-lowering properties

B vitamins, folic acid and saffron have depression-lowering properties. The B vitamins play a role in the production of neurotransmitters and support a good metabolism in the brain. When you have a lot of stress, a lot of vitamin B is consumed in the body and you need more of this vitamin.

Tyrosine and Tryptophan are needed to create happiness-enhancing substances

Tyrosine is a precursor of the happiness hormone norepinephrine and tryptophan is a precursor of serotonin. When you take food that contains these substances, more norepinephrine and serotonin are produced by the body.

Coffee, Alcohol and Smoking cause damage to the physical and to the energetic body

Coffee, alcohol and smoking have a degrading effect on the physical body. In addition, these substances also affect your energy body; they close you off more from spirituality. Also all three have a social function, which means that stopping these stimulants can be extra difficult and requires a lot of perseverance.

Coffee is the foundation of inner turmoil. This also applies to decaffeinated coffee and black tea, which also contain caffeine. Coffee stimulates the sympathetic nervous system, which brings you into a state of high activity. It does help your performance, but this is not really yours; it is caused by the adrenaline rush that your body experiences through the coffee. Because of the caffeine in your blood, it is very difficult to come to rest even hours later. This can cause sleep problems.

You should not suddenly stop coffee, because that is difficult for your nervous system to tolerate. However, you can gradually reduce it. That can initially give a feeling of emptiness.

Personally, I could never have imagined a life without coffee. However, what made me decide to stop was the fact that Fons Delnooz and Patricia Martinot described in their book *Voeding en Spiritualiteit [Food and Spirituality]* how coffee stands in the way of consciousness.

My life without coffee gives me much more peace, calm and balance. I no longer feel rushed and I now give in when I am tired by going to sleep for a while during the day.

Coffee is the foundation of inner turmoil

Alcohol causes your spiritual life to be crippled and you to lose your sense of responsibility for yourself. It affects your brain, liver and kidneys, and is a big polluter of the body, making you tired the next day because the body has to break down so much waste.

Smoking pollutes both the physical body and the energy bodies of man. Access to spirituality is reduced by smoking.

In the chapters on body-oriented therapy, physical exercise and in this chapter on nutrition I have spoken about individual factors that contribute to depression. However, depression is often the result of systemic factors; of things you carry from your family. This is the subject of the next chapter: 'Family Constellations'.

Part 4

Family Constellations

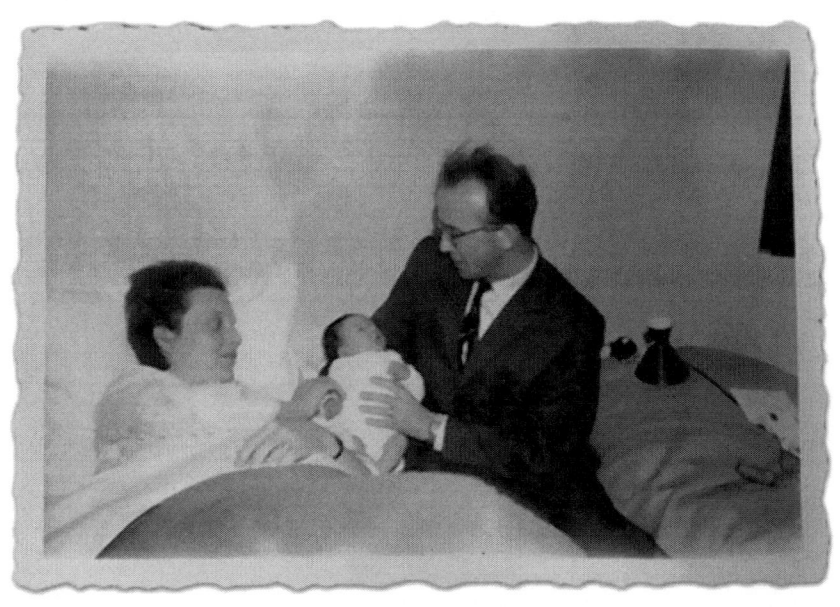

14 FAMILY CONSTELLATIONS

Becoming the child of your parents again

I have discovered something about true perfection. It starts with coming to terms with yourself. That is the first thing. Many people are inwardly torn apart, they are not satisfied with themselves. If you examine it, you can see that they have banned one of their parents or even both parents from their heart. Then they are cut off from the source of their lives. If someone is cut off from one of his parents, he has only half of his life force and if someone has only half of his life force, he becomes depressed. Depression is a feeling of emptiness, not of sadness. To have a feeling of emptiness means that one of the parents is missing. Then the heart is only half full. The depression disappears and someone comes to terms with himself, if he both honours and loves both parents. If this happens it is experienced as grace. I cannot just make up my mind to do this. If it succeeds, it is experienced as a gift. Then the basic feeling becomes lighter and more fulfilled and the depression is over. *

Bert Hellinger

---

* Bert Hellinger - *De Wijsheid is Voortdurend Onderweg [Wisdom is Continuously On the Way]*

In family constellations - a process developed by Bert Hellinger and which I will explain later in this chapter - we see that depression is often a part of something that is much larger than the person who has the depression.

The depression can arise for example because we may carry - out of love - the fate of someone in our family who didn't want to live any more, perhaps because that person wanted in turn to follow another person into death, again out of love. This all happens unconsciously.

Seeing such an entanglement within your family system makes it possible to get out of the identification you have with the other family member.

When the family member with whom you were identified is recognised and honoured, you feel in harmony and from that moment on this person gives you strength and support. Now you are free to lead your own life and are no longer determined by patterns that are not yours.

Depression is often part of something that is much bigger than the person who has the depression

---

Identification is an unconscious phenomenon; when someone from the family system is not recognised or appreciated, someone from a later generation takes over his or her role, to still ensure that this person is included. There appears to be an invisible 'law' in life that everyone is of equal value and significance and that everyone has the right to belong. This is not a theory in itself. It's something that shows experientially in the family constellations.

When you are depressed you can ask the question in a family constellation what lies behind the depression. You then come together with a group of people from amongst whom you choose individuals (representatives) to represent some of your family members. You also choose a representative for yourself. You position the representatives in the room according to your feeling, without giving them instructions. What you can then see is a portrait of your family that expresses something about the level of feelings of intimacy, pain, love or abandonment that the family members have in relation to each other.

When they are positioned in place, the representatives of the family members start feeling things that in reality the original family member feels or has felt. This is possible because we are all part of a large energy field, that is also called 'the great soul'. The representatives follow the impulses to move which arise in their body. This is not something they think about, but something that just happens, driven by the energy of the field in which they find themselves.

A facilitator leads the family constellation, tuning in to the energy field in which all representatives are present. He looks at the points when as a child your love was interrupted, and what can be done now to complete the original movement of outreach (in particular to the parents). In the end, where possible, a solution is found that feels right for all family members.

Bert Hellinger has discovered experientially (through the many family constellations he has facilitated) 'that depressions usually develop when one of the parents is excluded; if that parent has no place. For example, if the mother is excluded because she is sick. The child then takes care of the mother, instead of taking* the mother. In this way the mother has no active force in the heart of the child.'*

---

* Bert Hellinger - *De Wijsheid is Voortdurend Onderweg [Wisdom is Continuously On the Way]*

* Bert Hellinger describes 'taking' as follows: "When I take, I take what is available exactly as it is. This kind of taking is humble, and acknowledges the parents as they are. In taking I also acknowledge myself exactly as I am. It has a deep conciliatory quality - a coming to rest. It's beyond judgement of good or bad. Boasting about one's parents is also a sign of not having taken them. Idealizing shuts out the essential as well."*

---

*Depression mostly develops
when one of the parents is excluded*

When you don't take the parent you are not nourished and you cannot lead your own life; you keep looking back then to the parent, in an attempt to be able still to receive from him or her.

I recognize myself in the above. As a child, I wanted to carry the pain of my mother, who had had such traumatic experiences in the Japanese concentration camp. I therefore took the role of mother-of-my-mother which meant I didn't take her as mother and could not receive from her. In this way the void arose in me which was to become my depression.

In Meera Hashimoto's Art Therapist Training this becomes very clear to me in an exercise. Meera asks us to form groups of three people. The first of the three represents the child that you used to be, the second your mother and the third the fate of your mother. When it is my turn I myself represent the fate of my mother. The two others represent me-as-a-child and

---

* Bert Hellinger - *Acknowledging What Is*

my mother. Then we move without words, in whatever way our feeling guides us. Later we share with each other what each of us has felt.

The representative for me-as-a-child wants to go to the mother but is afraid and tiptoes very carefully around her all the time. The mother does not look at her fate. I represent in this constellation the fate of my mother, and feel that I am a Japanese from the concentration camp in which she had to stay as a child. As the fate-of-my-mother I feel the agitation of wanting to reach the mother, who doesn't look at me, and I feel irritated by the child. The child indicates later (when we share our experiences after the constellation), that she made an effort to get her mother to look at her fate. In the constellation the mother does all of a sudden look at her fate. As the representative of this fate, I feel an enormous anger towards the mother and grab her by the wrists, which I almost squeeze. The mother then feels that she cannot escape and she relaxes. I feel how the power of me-as-fate enters her. With this, I can let go of the mother and feel calm. The mother goes back to her child and takes her under her care. The child then rests with the mother.

Seeing and experiencing this is an important turnaround for me. Now I am grateful for the fate of my mother (that is, for the Japanese occupier) because I have seen and felt how much strength he has given her. It is courageous of me to dare to face this. Previously I have wanted to support my mother by rejecting the Japanese. In the place of blaming my mother as I did before in many therapies for what she had not given me, I now feel proud of her and of the fact that I am born to such a powerful woman. I am also proud of the child in me who made her look at her fate in this constellation. She didn't want this before because she wanted to focus totally on caring for me, but unless she looked at her fate she wasn't able to take care of me. I now see that she needed her fate to become strong. For this she had to go into the concentration camp. It was completely wrong of me to try as a child to take her fate away from her. It feels very good that I have seen in this constellation that my mother has owned the power of her destiny, and has taken this power into her body. Now I can rest in being-my-mother's-child and I can own my own destiny.

Now I can rest in being-my-mother's-child and I can own my own destiny

---

When I walk out of the group room, I meet - in my imagination - my mother. She stands in front of me next to the garden path on the Amalurra site. Next to her I see my father standing in his full height and strength. Very relaxed I stand before them as their child and look up to them. I feel safe and secure, with deep respect and gratitude for them. In the past I have sensed that my father felt helpless because he could not do anything for my mother with her pain. Because of this, to me he seemed to lack certain strength. Now that my mother has owned her own strength by accepting what has happened in the war, she has become available to my father and they are each present for me and together as powerful parents. Taking my parents gives me a feeling of self-worth; my parents are behind me now with their strength, and support me. That my parents have long since died is not important here; for me they are alive in the present. I can now turn around and focus on my own life path. For the first time in my life I experience a calm, content happiness and a deep relaxation.

Bert Hellinger names this happiness as one of the two ways we can experience happiness:

"If someone delivers good work, if he succeeds well in something and if what he does works well, then he becomes happy. This happiness feels like fulfillment, it is independent of the so-called 'feeling of happiness'. It has something essential, something full. It makes happy, even if you are in an unpleasant situation in which you are not happy.

"Then there is also the feeling of lightness; also this is happiness. I can have it with others together but also independently of them. This light-hearted feeling occurs when I have taken my parents, and when they live in me. And just as a whole, exactly as they are. Who takes his parents in this way, experiences that all the good that they have flows from them to you and that everything you feared or rejected in them remains outside. Who succeeds in this, notices how his sense of happiness grows."*

This last kind of happiness happens to me after this family constellation.

Svagito Liebermeister, husband of Meera Hashimoto, with whom I later train in family constellations, has written a book about family constellations called *'Roots of Love'*. I now feel personally what this title means: taking my parents in love gives me roots in the earth. For the first time in my life I feel really connected to the earth and I am grateful that I live on earth.

Svagito: 'You can only flower in your life when you feel that you have the best parents you could have. You cannot force this; it can only happen to you.'

---

* Bert Hellinger - *De wijsheid is voortdurend onderweg [Wisdom is Continuously On the Way]*

Taking my parents in love gives me roots in the earth

From a systemic point of view, there is harmony when everyone in the family system takes their proper role. This is not a rule or a theory, but something that shows itself in the family constellations. It is not easy to adopt the position of being the child again in relation to your parents when you have invested so many years in wanting to look after them; it has become part of your identity. You have to let go of your ego then. You have to be able to bow your head. At this point it can look like everything you stood for is gone without knowing what will happen instead. Sometimes several constellations are needed to take this step. Meditation is essential here, because meditation allows you to be able to stand alone in yourself.

A second thing that is difficult when letting go of the parental role you had adopted is that it is accompanied by guilt. The feeling of guilt arises from the fear of no longer belonging if you give up your caring role. Not to belong can be experienced as life-threatening. Here too meditation helps; it helps you to endure this guilt, which is inevitable.

When someone who is depressed feels he is entangled too much with his parents, he is often invited in a therapy situation to express his anger towards them. It is thought that this is a way to become free from one's parents. In his book *Acknowledging What Is* Bert Hellinger describes that in family constellations he sees that when someone does this, "he will punish himself for this. His self-punishment may be expressed in some kind of failure: in work, perhaps by losing a job or being unable to find work; or in relationships, by losing a partner; or by losing a lot of money.

"As a rule, someone is only depressed when he has not fully taken one of his parents. If someone expresses his anger in the way described above, he pushes the parent even further away, which can only lead to increased depression.

"Apart from taking care of one's parents, also demanding how they should be is a form of not taking and rejecting them. When a person makes demands about how his parents should be, or what his parents ought to do for him, it prevents him taking from them what is essential, by which he remains empty."*

> *When you demand how your parents should be, you remain empty*

Psychiatrist Gradus van Florestein, who works a lot with family constellations, says: "When we respect those with more experience, with more strength and wisdom than us, and know them to be behind us with their knowledge, strength and wisdom, then we live more fully and we are capable of more."**

Before asking for a family constellation, you don't have to know with which family member you are identified or where you have stepped into an inappropriate role. You can't know this, because it all happens unconsciously. It becomes visible by what you see happening before your eyes in the constellation. The seeing in itself is healing, because it helps you understand your own and your family members' situation.

---

* Bert Hellinger - *Acknowledging What Is*
** Gradus van Florestein - *De Depressie vanuit Verschuivend Perspectief [Depression from a Shifting Perspective]*

One constellation is often sufficient. You take in the image you see before you of the 'solution' - the establishment in which all family members feel harmonious - and that image often goes on working inside you for years. Hellinger says: "the soul goes slowly"; it is a process that needs time. You don't think about it anymore. The newly acquired insight will lead its own life.

In addition, body-oriented therapy may be needed, to work with the tensions that have settled in the body as a result of years of identification with another person or in adopting a wrong role within the household or within the family.

Meditation is indispensable for deepening and for being able to integrate the insights of the family constellation and essential for embarking on the journey into yourself. The next two chapters are about meditation.

Part 5

The Importance of Osho Meditations

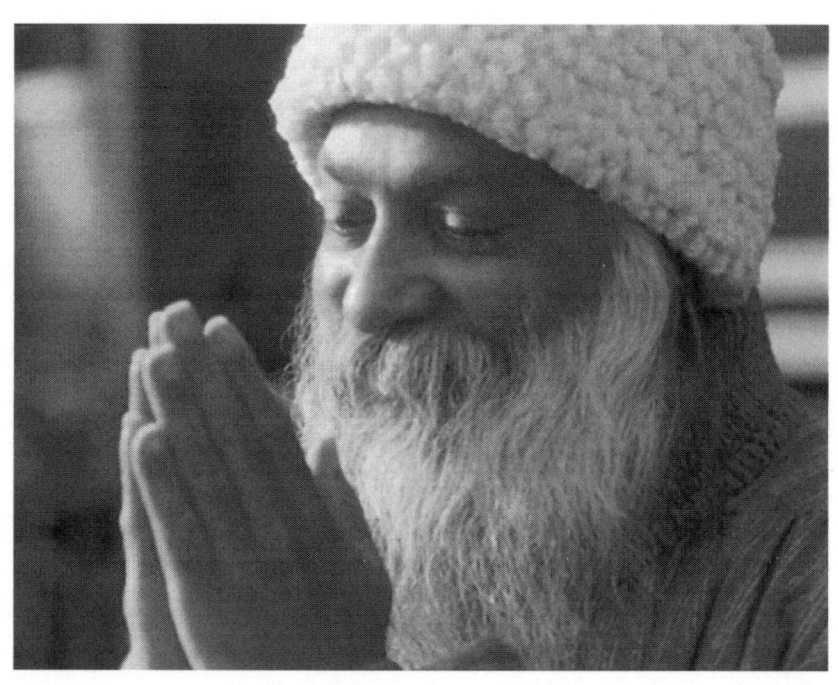

15 OSHO® ACTIVE MEDITATIONS

The mental alone won't do: the body has to be brought in it. That is why, in my meditation techniques, I do not take you as divided: you are one. If your mind is feeling angry, allow your body to be angry. If your mind is feeling happy, allow your body to dance. Do not create a division. Let yourself come deep down into the body and allow the body to flow to your innermost core. Become a flow!

You are frozen. I would like to melt you and create a flow again. That is why I insist on active meditation. By 'active' I only mean that your body must be involved in it. If you simply sit in a Buddha posture, you can go on thinking and thinking and thinking; the body is not involved in it. And the body is the world. Through the body you are related to the existence, through the body you exist. Your meditation must in some way be deeply rooted in the body; otherwise it will become just a dream floating in the mind, just like clouds without any roots in the earth. I want to push you back to the earth. *

Osho

---

* Osho - *The Supreme Doctrine #1*

Therapy cannot be the final treatment for depression. The mind is very inventive in constantly creating new problems and you can spend a lifetime working on solving these. Therapy is only successful if it is a preparation for meditation by removing the blockages that prevent it.

Therapy is only successful
if it is a preparation for meditation

Meditation creates a distance between you and the mind (thinking). When you meditate you become more and more aware of thoughts, feelings and emotions without identifying yourself with them. Finally, between all those thoughts and sensations there arise silences, which gradually grow bigger. When you are totally alert and aware, problems cannot occur anymore.

When you are totally alert and aware,
problems cannot arise any more

Osho, an Indian mystic, has made meditation accessible to the Western person who, living in such a speedy society and exposed to so much information and stimuli, finds it almost impossible to be silent inside as a result of all the disturbance experienced.

When somebody tries consciously to go inside, then they encounter all kinds of things inside themselves which they don't want to see: anger, agitation, sadness, hatred, jealousy and frustration. When they start sitting on a chair or meditation cushion with their eyes closed to meditate, they are sitting on a volcano of bubbling restlessness and haunting thoughts. If they try to push away those thoughts and feelings, they start hiding in their subconscious mind and from there they start causing disease, tensions and fear. The person may feel that they are going crazy, and that can actually happen if they don't find a way to express what is going on in them.

That is the reason that Osho has developed active meditations, in which space for expression is given in the first stages.

When you have first been able to give expression to what's inside of you, you will come to a state of rest and silence much easier

Osho: "Tensions have to be transformed, tensions have to be used in a creative way so that they don't destroy you - rather they create something.

"Something creative should be born out of your silence. So my emphasis is basically on active methods. Silence should come through activity, creativity - through painting, dance, music. It should remain continuously joined with action so it does not annihilate action; on the contrary it enhances it"*

I describe the original instructions of Osho for the Meditations and meditative processes in this chapter in the words of Osho himself - printed in italics.

I also reproduce literally the descriptions of Osho's Active Meditations and Meditative Therapies from the book *Osho - Meditation, the First and Last Freedom*, placed between these symbols: » «.

---

* Osho - *This Is It #7*

» All OSHO Active Meditations involve action - sometimes intense and physical, sometimes more gentle - followed by inaction, stillness. Some of the meditations are recommended for particular times of the day. All are accompanied by music that has been especially composed to support the different stages.

Audio and video instructions for the OSHO Active Meditations and other OSHO Meditations are given on osho.com/meditation and on imeditate.osho.com. For live participation options from your home, log in on: imeditate.osho.com.« *

Osho: "People ask me why I teach active meditations: it is the only way to find inaction.

Dance to the uttermost, dance in a frenzy, dance madly, and if your whole energy is involved in it, a moment comes when suddenly you see the dance is happening on its own - there is no effort in it. It is action without action."**

Active Meditations are the only way to find inaction

Osho emphasises that active meditations are only techniques, ones which help us to move our energy and create the space in which meditation can happen, but that the final meditation is a state of non-doing.

Osho: "The major part of life, the central part of life, should be like a happening. As the lightning happens in the clouds, so godliness happens. As rivers go on rushing towards the ocean and dissolve, so love happens. So happens meditation - it has nothing to do with your doing. Your doing is not

---

* Osho - *Meditation, the First and Last Freedom*
** Osho - *Meditation, the First and Last Freedom*

essential for it to happen. It can happen when you are sitting and not doing anything. In fact it happens only then, when you are not doing anything and you are sitting. I insist for you to do many things as methods, but the insistence is only this - that you have to be tired, otherwise you won't sit."*

Meditation is a happening; it has nothing to do with your doing

---

Psychiatrist Gradus van Florestein describes the importance of meditation in breaking the isolation experienced in depression:

"In meditation, you are no longer concerned with defining who you are; your 'I' and everything you do, your past and your future plans. That 'I' is a wave in the ocean of life and is one with this. In meditation you experience that you are part of this ocean. That you are not only the wave of the 'I' but at the same time the entire ocean. It is difficult to express in words. And yet it is so important in depression. When you're depressed, you're cut off from this unity. You are isolated from the existence around you and from the soul within yourself."**

In meditation you experience that you are part of the ocean of life

---

For me the most healing active meditation of Osho's is the Dynamic Meditation.

---

* Osho - *The Discipline of Transcendence*, Vol 2, #9
** Gradus van Florestein - *De Depressie vanuit Verschuivend Perspectief* [*Depression from a Shifting Perspective*]

OSHO® DYNAMIC MEDITATION

First, recognise your personality, and then break it.

My meditation technique is a system to break down your personality. It is not meditation but the removal of your personality. And once it is removed, meditation is a very natural thing. Once the rock is removed, you don't have to do anything to make the spring flow. The spring flows by itself; it is only a question of removing the stone.

Meditation is your nature. If the rock of your personality is not there, it will come automatically. But at least you should let something there be natural. Whether it is tears, or laughter, or dancing - at least let something natural happen. Then what is supremely natural is also bound to happen.*

Osho

When depressed, you are flat, grey and without energy. Under this grey layer a lot of emotions are hidden - especially anger and sadness - which have been suppressed in an earlier stage of life out of a survival strategy. It seems as if you have no emotions, while in fact they are present deep inside; compressed under the protective layer of the depression. When these emotions can be discharged or felt with consciousness, liberation takes place and the depression cannot continue.

Under the depression emotions like anger and sadness are hidden

---

* Osho - *The Voice of Silence* #14

After my schema therapy of more than a year, when I start the twenty-one day 'Art Therapist Training' of Meera Hashimoto in Amalurra, it is also the beginning of twenty-one days Osho Dynamic Meditation; an active meditation, which I explain later in this chapter.

Everything that comes up in therapies can only be integrated in meditation; it is through meditation the insights happen.

Everything that comes up in therapies can only be integrated in meditation

In this training I get up early every morning and walk through the rising mists to the meditation room. I am determined to give everything I have in this meditation. I want to get out of this bleakness. It's now or never. And then, on the third day, when the last note of the meditation music has faded away and I am lying on my stomach on the floor to feel my body, there is life; flowing, lively and powerful. My body is filled with energy and in a dancing way I walk back to the hotel, my feet firmly connected to the earth. In the large wall mirror in the hotel hallway I see reflected what I have already felt inside: the light in my eyes is back. The people of my training group also see it: I shine.

The light in my eyes is back; I shine

Gratefully I run into the field of Amalurra and dance in the morning sun. I let myself fall on my stomach with my arms and legs stretched out in the dewy grass. For the first time in my life I feel connected to the earth and I want to live on this planet. I also feel now that I can let my unborn twin sister go. It is all right for me now that she is somewhere else in the universe and I cry out to her: 'I'm alive, I want to live!'

Then I make a promise to myself: I will continue this meditation every day, also when I am back home. I no longer want to consider something that is valuable to me as merely an accidental event that fades away a little later. And I stick to that promise; back home I wake up every morning at six o'clock to do this meditation as the first thing at the beginning of the day. I feel lively and light all day then because I am released from a lot of emotional ballast and I am better able to wait and to bear things. The meditation gives me more and more happiness and inner peace.

The Osho Dynamic Meditation gives me more and more happiness and inner peace

---

Instructions for the Dynamic Meditation
» This meditation is a fast, intense and thorough way to break old, ingrained patterns in the bodymind that keep one imprisoned in the past and to experience the freedom, the witnessing, silence and peace that are hidden behind those prison walls.

The meditation is meant to be done in the early morning, when "the whole of nature becomes alive, the night has gone, the sun is coming up and everything becomes conscious and alert."

You can do this meditation alone, but to start with, it can be helpful to do it with other people. It is an individual experience, so remain oblivious of others around you. Wear loose, comfortable clothing.

This meditation is to be done with its specific OSHO Dynamic Meditation music, which indicates and energetically supports the different stages. This music you can get from all spiritual bookstores and on www.osho.com.

The meditation lasts one hour and has five stages. Keep your eyes closed throughout, using a blindfold if necessary.

This is a meditation in which you have to be continuously alert, conscious, aware, whatsoever you do. Remain a witness. And when - in the fourth stage - you have become completely inactive, frozen, then this alertness will come to its peak.« *

First stage: 10 minutes

Breathing chaotically through the nose, let the breathing be intense, deep, fast, without rhythm, with no pattern - and concentrating always on the exhalation. The body will take care of the inhalation. The breath should move deeply into the lungs. Do this as fast and as hard as you possibly can, until you literally become the breathing. Use your natural body movements to help you to build up your energy. Feel it building up, but don't let go during the first stage.

Second stage: 10 minutes

EXPLODE! Let go of everything that needs to be thrown out. Follow your body. Give your body freedom to express whatever is there. Go totally mad. Scream, shout, cry, jump, kick, shake, dance, sing, laugh; throw yourself around. Hold nothing back; keep your whole body moving. A little acting often helps to get

---

* Osho - *Meditation: the First and Last Freedom*

you started. Never allow your mind to interfere with what is happening. Consciously go mad. Be total.

Third stage: 10 minutes

With arms raised high above your head, jump up and down shouting the mantra "Hoo! Hoo! Hoo!" as deeply as possible. Each time you land on the flats of your feet, let the sound hammer deep into the sex center. Give all you have: exhaust yourself completely.

Fourth stage: 15 minutes

STOP! Freeze wherever you are, in whatever position you find yourself. Don't arrange the body in any way. A cough, a movement, anything, will dissipate the energy flow and the effort will be lost. Be a witness to everything that is happening to you.

Fifth stage: 15 minutes

Celebrate! With music and dance, express whatsoever is there. Carry your aliveness with you throughout the day. *

» Note: If your meditation space prevents you from making noise, you can do this silent alternative: rather than throwing out the sounds, let the catharsis in the second stage take place entirely through bodily movements. In the third stage, the

---

*   Osho - *Meditation: the First and Last Freedom*

sound Hoo! can be hammered silently inside and the fifth stage can become an expressive dance.

This is a meditation in which you have to be continuously alert, conscious, aware, whatsoever you do. Remain a witness. Don't get lost. «*

It is good to do the meditation at least seven days in a row. Then a cycle in yourself is complete. Twenty-one days is an even more complete cycle.

The muscle pain that often occurs, certainly in the first days, is not only caused by the intense movements but also because blockages are coming loose. When you continue with the meditation the pain usually disappears and a flow starts happening in the previously painful parts of the body.

---

*In this meditation
blockages in the body are coming loose*

The Dynamic Meditation is a contradiction. 'Dynamic' means effort, much effort, absolute effort, and 'meditation' means silence, no effort, no activity. You can call it a dialectical meditation.

Osho says about this:

"Be so active that the whole energy becomes a movement; no energy is left static in you. The whole energy has been called forth, nothing is left behind. All the frozen parts of energy are melting, flowing. You are not a frozen thing now, you have become dynamic. You are not like substance now, you are more like energy. You are not material, you have become

---

* Osho - *Meditation: the First and Last Freedom*

electrical. Bring total energy to work, to be active, moving.

When everything is moving and you have become a cyclone, then become alert. Remember, be mindful - and in this cyclone suddenly you will find a centre which is absolutely silent. This is the centre of the cyclone. This is you - you in your divinity, you as a god.

All around you is activity. Your body has become an active cyclone - everything moving fast, faster. All the frozen parts have melted, you are flowing. You have become a volcano, fire, electricity.

But just in the centre, amidst all this movement, there is a non-moving point, the still point.

This still point is not to be created. It is there, you are not to do anything about it. It has always been there. It is your very being, the very ground of your being. This is what Hindus have been calling the atman, the soul. It is there, but unless your body, unless your material existence becomes totally active, you will not be aware of it. With total activity the totally inactive becomes apparent. The activity gives you a contrast. It becomes the blackboard, and on the blackboard is the white dot. On a white wall you cannot see a white dot; on a blackboard the white dot appears to you.

So when your body has become active, dynamic, a movement, suddenly you become aware of a point which is still, absolutely still - the unmoving centre of the whole moving world. That is effortless. No effort is made for it. No effort is needed, it is simply revealed. Effort on the part of the periphery, no effort on the part of the centre. Movement on the periphery, stillness at the centre. Activity on the periphery, absolute inactivity at the centre.

Effort and effortlessness, movement and no movement, activity and no activity, matter and the soul - these are the banks. And between these two banks flows the invisible. These two banks are visible. Between these two flows the invisible. That you are."*

Effort and effortlessness, these are the banks. Between these banks flows the invisible - which is you

---

In the next chapter I describe three Meditative Therapies of Osho: processes of one or three weeks, which although they work as a therapy are meditations.

---

* Osho - *My Way: The Way of the White Clouds* #4

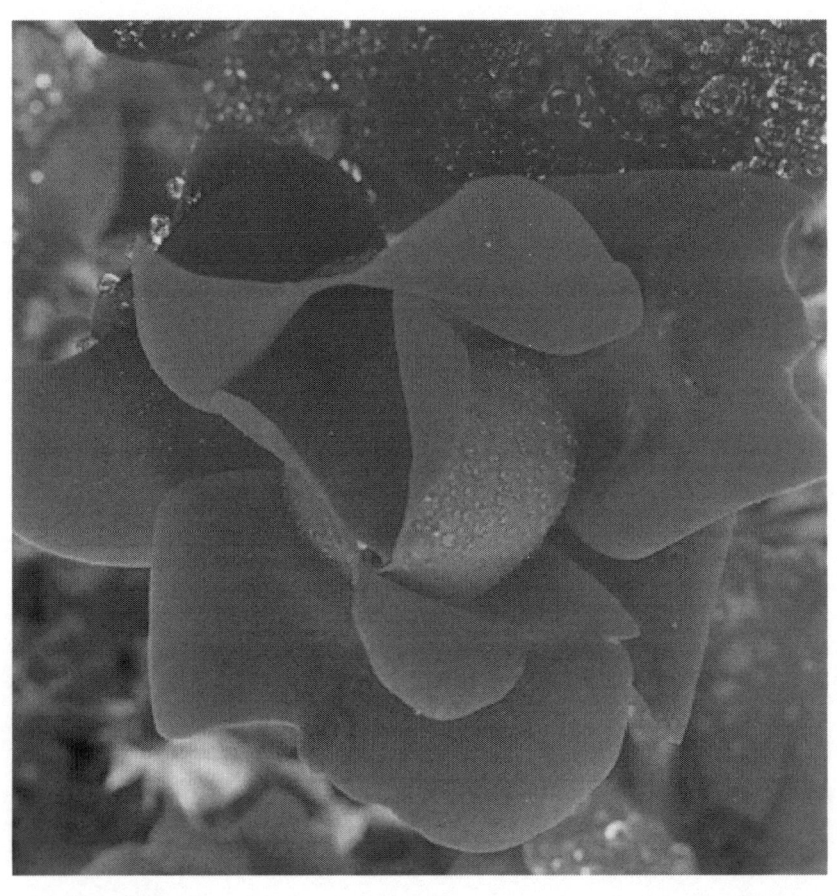

16 OSHO® MEDITATIVE THERAPIES

It is your very nature to be blissful. Meditation gives you only that which you have always had. It simply makes you aware of your reality. It does not bring in anything new. It simply reveals to you the treasure that is lying there ignored and neglected, while you are running all over the world for it. You will not find it anywhere else because it is within you.*

Osho

Apart from the Active Meditations, Osho has created four Meditative Therapies, three of which I mention in this book: the Osho® Mystic Rose, the Osho® Born Again and the self-hypnosis process Osho® Reminding Yourself of the Forgotten Language of Talking to Your BodyMind.

» The first two are radical expressive processes that lead to a final stage of silent self-awareness. Uniquely simple and effective, these energetic methods involve a minimum of interaction among the participants, but the energy of the group and

---

*   Osho - *Meditation, the First and Last Freedom*

the presence of a trained facilitator help each individual go more deeply into his or her own process.

Osho® Reminding Yourself of the Forgotten Language of Talking to Your BodyMind is a guided process for activating the self-healing powers of the bodymind and for making friends with oneself.

Osho Meditative Therapies are offered regularly at the Osho International Meditation Resort in Pune, India and at larger Osho Meditation Centres worldwide. Once you have participated in the group process, you can continue the method alone at home whenever you like. «*

The meditative therapies do work as a therapy, but they are essentially meditations; they work outside of your mind. They ensure that you can free yourself from old, fixed patterns, that you regain your vitality and that space is created in you for meditation.

They are energetic processes, that form a direct connection from yourself to yourself.

The Meditative Therapies of Osho work outside of the mind; they form a direct connection from yourself to yourself

---

* Osho - *Meditation, the First and Last Freedom*

OSHO® MYSTIC ROSE

Laughter and Crying connect you with your *being*

All that this world needs is a good cleansing of the heart and all the inhibitions of the past. Laughter and tears can do both. Tears will take out all the agony that is hidden inside you and laughter will take all that is preventing your ecstasy. Once you have learned the art you will be immensely surprised: why has this not been told up to now? There is a reason: nobody has wanted humanity to have the freshness of a rose flower and the fragrance and the beauty. *

Osho

When I am depressed I try to get out of my head through my head and that doesn't work. The connection with my being is broken.

Osho explains that if you want to go from your head into your being, the heart is an intermediate station. The Osho Mystic Rose is a process that opens your heart, gives you the chance to cry out the sadness that is hidden under the depression and leads you to your own ecstasy and inner silence.

---

*   Osho - *Yaa Hoo! The Mystic Rose* #30

When I visit the Osho International Meditation Resort in Pune (India) for the first time in January 1995, I become fascinated by the eyes of people who are wearing a badge on which a rose is depicted. Their eyes are like still water; pure, clear and with an immense depth.

The eyes of the people who do the Osho Mystic Rose look like a deep, silent lake with an immense depth

---

I find out that these people are doing the Osho Mystic Rose; a meditative therapy created by the Indian Mystic Osho. I don't ask any further. Because I long for such beautiful eyes I register for this process, my experiences of which I will describe later in this chapter.

Instructions from Osho for the Osho Mystic Rose:

'The Mystic Rose is a three-week process, lasting three hours per day. During the first week you laugh, for no reason at all, dissolving the layers of dust, inhibitions and repressions that prevent inner spontaneity and joy. The second week is devoted to weeping and crying for no reason at all - allowing the pain and the tears that are ready to come and which we have been preventing. The third week is for silence and stillness - the watcher on the hills - silent watching, meditation.' *

Three hours a day are needed, because a dam in us has to be broken.

---

*   Osho - *Meditation, the First and Last Freedom*

» The symbol of the mystic rose is that, if man takes care of the seed that he is born with, gives it the right soil, gives it the right atmosphere and the right vibrations, moves on a right path where the seed can start growing. Then the ultimate growth is symbolised as the mystic rose - when your being blossoms and opens all its petals and releases a beautiful fragrance. «*

Osho: "When a man reaches his innermost being he will find the first layer is of laughter and the second layer is of agony, tears.

"If you cry and weep without any reason, just as an exercise, a meditation, nobody will believe it. Tears have never been accepted as a meditation. And I tell you, they are not only a meditation, they are a medicine also. You will have better eyesight and you will have a better inner vision."**

Osho on the Mystic Rose:

"All that this world needs is a good cleansing of the heart, of all the inhibitions of the past. Laughter and tears can do both. Tears will take out all the agony that is hidden inside you and laughter will take all that is preventing your ecstasy. Once you have learned the art you will be immensely surprised: Why has this not been told up to now? There is a reason: nobody has wanted humanity to have the freshness of a rose flower and the fragrance and the beauty."***

---

*   Osho - *Meditation, the First and Last Freedom*
** Osho - *Meditation, the First and Last Freedom*
*** Osho - *Meditation, the First and Last Freedom*

> "Your heart is the soil
> Your trust is the climate
> And your being is the mystic rose -
> which is opening, blossoming, releasing its fragrance.
>
> The mystic rose is just a symbol of the man
> whose being is dormant no more,
> is asleep no more, but is fully awake
> and has opened all its petals and
> has become sensitive to all that is truthful, beautiful, good -
> the very splendor of existence."*

My first Mystic Rose in 1995 in the Osho International Meditation Resort in Pune, India

First week: the week of Laughter

One hundred and twenty people assemble in a big group room. After a short explanation about laughing without any reason, jumping happily in the air we shout 'Yahoo' three times and start laughing. It is a colourful mixture of sounds. The fake-laugh of the very beginning, the exuberant laughter as spontaneous laughter arises out of nowhere, laughter because I suddenly see a so-cute Chinese face behind all the one hundred and twenty other people, laughter because I remember a funny incident or just laughter about something that should be seen as sad.

Time exists no more, because we had to leave our watches behind. From the level of the water in the two bottles I brought (as

---

* Osho - *Yaa Hoo! The Mystic Rose* #30

fuel for the laughter) I see a little bit how the time is progressing. I get muscle pain in my jaws. It is so funny. It doesn't matter what work somebody does, where they come from or what their age is; there is only laughter.

Time exists no more; there is only the laughter

By the seventh day, three hours laughing is no longer enough. In the lunch break I am lying on my back on a small table under a tree, laughing out loud from pure delight; because of the green of the tree, my body, which is so alive, the humour of everyday life and the way a fly moves its legs when it is walking over the table. Slowly, slowly people are gathering around me, joining in the laughter, more and more, for no reason at all - until long after the lunch is over.

In this week there is no crying. Osho has separated laughter and crying in this process. If you feel tempted to cry, you have to turn it into laughter.

During the week of laughter we automatically come closer to our tears.

Second week: the week of Crying

Day eight: the pink bedsheets of the mattresses have been changed into staid blue. Everyone has a bedsheet to cover him- or herself and a box of tissues next to the blue pillow. Silently everyone enters. We have opened ourselves to our pain, our wounds, and not only to the tears we did not cry but also to the tears of gratefulness and being touched.

A little bit uneasy and silent we sit down on our mattresses. After a short invitation to open ourselves to our pain, we quietly say "Yaboo" three times and lie down and start making soft whimpering sounds to help ourselves start to cry. In some corners it is silent. In other corners people start sobbing softly.

Soon the space is filled with sadness and pain. Some people can cry easily, while others are struggling with their inhibitions. Sometimes there is sad music for a while.

Slowly, slowly I drop my resistance to crying in the presence of others while still protecting myself carefully with my bedsheet, not to be seen. Things that I had never known had been so painful for me as a child come up, like the loss of a primary school friend and something scary in the baby stroller. I feel I am recognising profoundly something very deep inside of me. What I am feeling feels so true, far more than any theories I ever created in my life about myself and my past. It feels more authentic than any psychotherapist's analysis ever. This is something which is so direct; a direct connection from myself to myself.

There is nobody who tells me to stop crying. There is no-one who consoles me, to take away my sadness. Yet at the same time there is so much consolation: the presence of all the others around me, who also took the courage to bring into the daylight everything which is buried most deep inside of us and to heal it in this way. When I cry about something and someone else is also crying, it feels like the other person is crying with me and sharing my sorrow. And this is healing. So many times I have been crying alone and felt so lonely in it. And now: we are doing it together, even though everyone lies apart from each other on their own mattress, with a space in between.

> *There is no-one who consoles me to take away my sadness and at the same time the presence of the others is so consoling*

At the end of the last hour on the last day of crying, I feel a gentle hand on my shoulder. I look up and somebody is standing in front of me with the most beautiful rose I have ever seen. I cry; out of being deeply touched and out of gratitude. This rose is the recognition of all the tears I have cried and of all the joy I have expressed in the laughter. It is the recognition of the rose I carry in my heart and which has opened its petals. By the laughter and crying the beautiful fragrance of my inner rose is released. And I see my tears reflected in the small drops of water on the deep red petals, which shine towards me like pearls. We hug each other with the rose in our hands.

Third week: Witnessing in Silence

Grateful, we enter the third stage: 'the watcher on the hill'. The stage of witnessing. With closed eyes we sit three quarters of an hour in silence on our meditation cushion, watching everything that is happening inside us; remnants of sadness, waves of anger, thoughts, serene silence, a tendency to laugh. Moment after moment all of this is changing.

After three quarters of an hour there is an opportunity to dance in a soft way, standing on the spot, so we can both keep focused on ourselves and move our body at the same time. And then again we sit for forty-five minutes. In this way (sitting, followed by fifteen minutes of dance) we complete our three hours of witnessing. When I open my eyes after three hours and leave the group room, it is a magnificent experience. Nature enters straight in my heart; so pure, with such tremendously beautiful colours. Everything is surrounded by silence. It feels as if a haze, which has always been before my eyes, has suddenly disappeared; as if my glasses, which were always fogged, have been cleaned. My walking is like a dance and I hug my friends; friends whom I had avoided during the crying stage because I felt so vulnerable. I feel a tremendous joy. A celebration of life, in myself and with others.

I look in the mirror and I see mystic rose eyes! The eyes I was longing for when I started the process.

Nature enters straight in my heart.
Everything is surrounded by silence

I almost can't describe in words what the Osho Mystic Rose has brought me. It has opened something in me that has nothing to do with words. I have become more authentic; I have come into contact with what is pure in me. I feel confirmed in what really matters; something that has nothing to do with performance, studies or ambitions. I have felt my real joy and laugh a lot more about everything around me; see the laughable in so many small things. I have felt what has really made me sad and how important it is to release through tears that sadness. I have been amazed at everything in myself and around me in the beautiful silence of the third week. Now I only look for what corresponds to what is real and pure, in myself and around me.

By the Osho Mystic Rose I have become more authentic

In the years that follow I do the Mystic Rose again many times, once all by myself. It is possible to do it this way too, but not good for the first time when it is necessary to go through the process with a facilitator and in a group. I also follow the Osho Mystic Rose training in Pune, in order to be able to facilitate this process.

I have experienced how the Mystic Rose has taken me out of my depression and I am grateful when I see that happening as well to participants in the Mystic Rose groups I facilitate. Participants who have started the Mystic Rose being depressed get back the colour on their cheeks and their eyes start shining more. At the end of the process they tell me that they are no longer depressed.

OSHO® BORN AGAIN

In the flow by connecting with your inner child

Just be soft, flowing. Be like a child and always retain the purity and the softness of childhood. Don't lose contact with it and you will be surprised one day when you discover that the child that you had been fifty years before is still alive within you.

If you know how to make contact with it, suddenly you are again a child; the child is never lost because that is your life. It remains there; it is not that the child dies and then you become young and then the youth dies, then you become old; no!

Layers upon layers accumulate but the innermost core remains the same, the babe that you were born is still there within you; many layers have accumulated around it - if you penetrate those layers, suddenly the child explodes in you; this explosion I have called 'ecstasy'. *

Osho

In my depression my life flow has become blocked. I have lost the connection with my being and thus also with my inner child, which is the core of my being.

Dark thoughts about the past and the future have gained the upper hand and it seems as if there is nothing left of the

---

* Osho - *Talking Tao #7*

energetic, pure, lively, authentic child in me that came into the world with such originality.

---

*In my depression I have lost the connection
with my inner child*

Osho: "My insistence on being playful is because of this: I want you to go back to the very point from where you stopped growing. There has been a point in your childhood when you stopped growing and when you started being false. You may have been angry, a small child in a tantrum, angry, and your father or your mother said, "Don't be angry! This is not good!" You were natural but a division was created and a choice was there for you. If you were to remain natural then you would not have got the love of your parents. Of course, you wanted the love; that was the only security for you, you could not have existed without it. So you opted, you surrendered. You pushed your nature aside. You started laughing and smiling; you became a good boy or good girl. The day you became the good boy or a good girl was the day of catastrophe. From that moment you have never been natural. From that moment you have been serious, never playful. From that moment you have been dying, not alive. From that moment you have been aging, not maturing."*

---

*The day you became the good boy or a good girl
was the day of catastrophe*

---

* *Osho - The Supreme Doctrine #1*

Instructions from Osho for the Born Again

"This is a one-week process, lasting two hours per day.

For the first hour you behave like a child, just enter your childhood. Whatever you wanted to do, do it - dancing, singing, jumping, crying, weeping - anything at all, in any posture. Nothing is prohibited except touching other people. Don't touch or harm anyone else in the group.

For the second hour just sit silently. You will be fresher, more innocent and meditation will become easier." *

What the Born Again has given me

For me, this process has restored in me the feeling of how it is to follow my flow of life from moment to moment without setting any goal. I have come to feel what makes me happy, what makes me excited and also what makes me sad or lonely.

I have also started to remember the child that I was and see that as an adult essentially the same things that made me happy as a child still warm me.

In this process I have also had the chance to express things that I did not have the chance to do as a child; for example, I screamed long and loudly, even though I could still hear voices in the background of my mind saying things like 'don't make so much noise, there are other people too'. I have started to be less concerned with what people think of me and to take more space for what I think is important. The process has made my meditation easier, because it has opened me to 'being with what is'.

---

*   Osho - *Meditation, the First and Last Freedom*

*The Osho® Born Again has opened me for meditation;
for 'being with what is'*

For a few years I have been facilitating the Osho® Born Again in Eindhoven. I see people becoming more alive throughout this process. They feel what the quality of the inner child is that they carry within them again; for some, that child is wild and outgoing, for others silent and contemplative. We carry many types of child in us: the frightened, shy, sad, happy, quiet, thoughtful, anxious, wild and naughty child. These all get space in this process.

There are also people who after experiencing Born Again have suddenly felt what the kind of work they want to do is and who have gone a totally different direction in their lives.

OSHO® REMINDING YOURSELF OF THE FORGOTTEN LANGUAGE OF TALKING TO YOUR BODYMIND

Healing from the Unconscious

Right now, when you find body, mind and heart in disharmony, first listen to the body. None of the so-called saints will say this to you. First listen to the body. The body has a wisdom of its own, and the body is uncorrupted by the priests; the body is unpolluted by your teachers, by your education, by your parents. Begin with the body, because right now the body is the purest thing in you. So if the heart and the mind go against it, let them go. You follow the body. The body is the first harmony and the being is the last. The fight is always between the heart and the head. The body and being are never in conflict - they are both natural. The body is visible nature and the being is invisible nature, but they are part of one phenomenon. *

Osho

During my periods of depression I am ashamed of having a body, since I am doing nothing meaningful with it; I do not know for what purpose my body is in this life. I am afraid to die before I have even lived with some inspiration.

---

* Osho - *The Rebellious Spirit* #22

Without feeling any connection with my body I take care of it routinely and without love; I automatically take a shower, carelessly cram my clothes in the washing machine, eat the same food every day without tasting it and look disapprovingly in the mirror at a face that I cannot love.

I am not aware of how loyal my body is to me. Despite my sombre mood my heart goes on beating, my lungs are breathing, my intestines digest my food, my bladder collects my urine, my bones carry me and my muscles keep me upright. In my depression there is not a trace of gratitude within me for all this.

The self-hypnosis process of Osho: Reminding Yourself of the Forgotten Language of Talking to your Bodymind, which I will describe below, has helped me to establish a friendly connection with my body and to listen to my body, to appreciate it and to understand its messages.

This Self-hypnosis process establishes a friendly, respectful connection with my body

---

Description of the process

» This is a guided one-week process, lasting one hour per day. It can then be continued and refreshed at any time.

The method is based on the understanding that we need to be taught anew to create friendship with our bodies and minds; these are not separate from us or from one another. We need to remember 'the forgotten language' of communicating with the bodymind about those areas where our tensions and pains exist.

In a light trance, while combining deep relaxation with alertness, you learn to harness the bodymind's creative and self-healing energies. These can be brought to any specific issues of imbalance or unease, such as smoking, eating imbalances, insomnia, aches and pain - any functions that are normally part of the body and which need to be brought to wholeness and balance again.

The seven-day process is offered at the Osho International Meditation Resort in Pune, India, and in a number of Osho centres.
The method is also available in many languages as a one-hour guided process, accompanied by its specific music which energetically supports the different stages. The music is available on www.osho.com. «*

I have not learned friendliness towards my body

Friendliness towards and contact with my body is something which I forgot early in my childhood. Many things have contributed to this: my mother's message that I didn't know what hunger was, the message of the church that your body is already sinful from the moment that Eve took a bite of the apple from the forbidden tree, the message of the fashion industry which promotes the slimming-ideal and of magazines that show bodies in sizes you can never match, the message of the gyms that unless you do a workout five times a week, your body cannot be fit, and even my medical studies which considered the body only as an efficient tool to be mechanically repaired by surgery and medicines if it doesn't function properly.

---

*   Osho - *Meditation, the First and Last Freedom*

*Early in my childhood I have unlearned friendliness
and I have lost the connection with my body*

My experience with this process

When I arrive at the Osho International Meditation Resort in Pune in a depressed state, I plan to be rigorous with myself. I assume that the more intense and painful the exercises in a therapy group are, the better.

To my surprise however, I become attracted to something completely different.

One morning I step, together with ten others, into a room with a soft pink carpet, with mattresses and soft pillows, where the self-hypnosis process Osho® Reminding Yourself of the Forgotten Language of Talking to your Bodymind is offered.

Just gentleness and friendliness create the healing conditions in this process.

For one week we lie on a mattress every morning and listen to the voice of the person who facilitates this process. By repeatedly pronouncing the word 'Osho' (which you can replace with the word 'Yes' if you don't have a connection with Osho), we enter into a trance in which we make contact with the subconscious mind, from which the healing takes place.

If we had consciously been able to do something about our symptoms (pain, fatigue, migraines, wrong eating habits, depression), we would have done it long before. But usually the cause of all this is in the subconscious. Ninety percent of us is unconscious. The subconscious mind is the most intelligent part in us, which takes care of our breathing, blood circulation, digestion, the healing of our wounds and of many other vital processes.

'Reminding yourself of the forgotten language' is phrased in this way because the contact with our subconscious was still with us when we were born. At that time we were still totally connected to ourselves. If we were hungry, we cried until we were fed. If we felt sleepy we slept, and if we wanted to scream we did so. When we grew up we started to impose more and more inhibitions on ourselves to satisfy our educators. We had to do this, because we were dependent on them for care and love.

Now in this process we are approaching our subconscious again for healing. That is only possible in an environment of relaxation and of doing nothing. Our conscious mind doesn't have to do anything.

In the beginning we establish the connection with those body parts which are calling our attention, by saying these sentences out loud: 'I want to come closer to you and be your friend. I have never thought about it that you have been working for me all these years and I have never thanked you. Is there anything I can do better for you in the future?'

---

*'I want to come closer to you and be your friend.
I have never thought about it that you have been working for me all these years and I have never thanked you.
Is there anything I can do better for you in the future?'*

The sentences touch me right away, because they are so loving and warm. I immediately feel that by speaking them I come very close to my body.

When we have pronounced the sentences we listen, look and sense what image, sentence or feeling comes up in us. Even if nothing comes up, the process works deep inside our subconscious.

We then connect with the guardian, who resides in our unconscious part. This guardian always has the best intentions for us. Our symptom (the depression for example) is the best that our guardian can provide us with at this moment. To understand this better, I give the following example:

If because we want to finish today a hole we have been digging all day in the garden and we have ignored the pain in our back, it may be that we suddenly have an attack of lumbago. This means we can no longer move forward or backward. Our body warned us many times before to stop digging because the pain in our back was increasing, but we didn't listen. Then comes the point when the guardian sees no alternative but to give us lumbago, so that we have to stop. Often what we do is start to complain about the pain in our back, rather than listening to what the guardian indicates.

In this self-hypnosis process we ask the guardian what his message is for us.

The guardian always has the best intentions for us

We then invite the guardian to connect with the creativity in us and to create - together with that creativity - three new ways that are better for us, and to test them in our daily lives.

During this self-hypnosis week I notice already how much I start taking care of my body in a very natural way. Without having to make any effort I pull something warm on when it's cold, throw away food that is unhealthy for me and take rest when I am tired.

I suddenly start doing things which I already knew were healthy without even thinking.

It comes from within, from a responsiveness and a softness and from a deep connection with my body. I feel now that my body is my friend and I have a deep respect for its loyalty and for its intelligent functioning.

Now I listen to the messages which the symptoms of my body and of unpleasant habits send me, and they suddenly turn out to be useful signals.

My body has always been loyal to me. Now I also want to stay loyal to my body; I want to feed it with the right food - to dress it with appropriate clothing for the temperature of the year - to let the joints flow by moving and dancing and to sleep enough to give it rest. My body has become my temple.

My body has always been loyal to me;
now I want also to be loyal to my body

I am grateful to Osho, who found this meditative process with the Tibetans and then adapted it to the current form. I am also grateful to myself, because I have allowed myself to approach my body in a soft, welcoming way and thus have re-established my connection with it again.

My desire, as well as being connected to my body, is also to be connected with others. This is the subject of the next chapter.

Part 6

Re-establishment of the Connection with Yourself and the Other

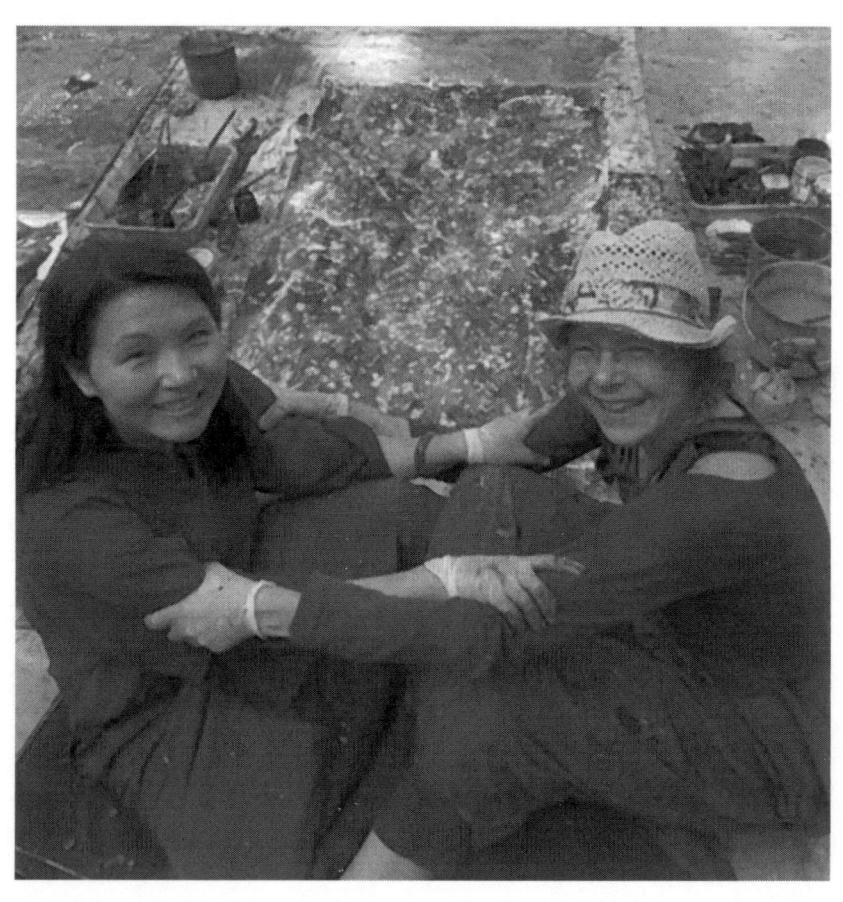

17 BEING CONNECTED AND IN CONTACT WITH THE OTHER

*If you love others, if your love is focused on others, you will live in darkness. Turn your light towards yourself first, become a light unto yourself first. Let the light dispel your inner darkness, you inner weakness. Let love make you a tremendous power, a spiritual force.**

*Osho**

I found it very difficult, if not impossible, to love myself when I was depressed. I found my life worthless because I could not find my passion and therefore could not flower. From this feeling-myself-worthless every connection with another person seemed to be pointless.

I loved my Indian partner very much, even though in essence you cannot love someone if you don't love yourself. What did I do in that case? I saw in him everything I could not find in myself: the way he lived in the here-and-now, his enthusiasm,

---

* Osho - *The Dhammapada: The Way of the Buddha*, Vol 5 #5

his friendliness, his humour, his rich social life, his meditation and his devotion to Osho. I adored him and put myself to one side for him. I was blind to his shortcomings and his limitations. When he did something that hurt me I blamed myself and looked inside for what I could do to open myself again to him.

You can only love someone if you love yourself

It is not that my love for my partner was fake; now that I am out of my depression I still love him very much, but in a healthier way. Now I see both his strong, light side and his injured, dark side. Now I will take a step back or give a response if necessary. As a result, our friendship has become less symbiotic and more the playing together of two individuals rooted in themselves. This only became possible by loving myself.

Family constellations were very important in starting to love myself, since they made it possible for me to take the position of 'the child of my parents' again and begin to reconnect with the love they have for me through which I have started to feel gratitude for the life they have given me.

Not being able to receive from another

In my depression I was out of touch with myself and therefore also out of touch with others. Yet nonetheless I went to my sisters as much as possible; I was terrified to be alone.

When I was with them it seemed for a while that I had a part in their lives, as if their cosiness was my cosiness and as if their children belonged to me too. But then, at home on my own again, I realised that being with my sisters had only increased the gap which I felt stretched between what they already had and everything I thought I still had to achieve, and panic struck me.

Even though my sisters wanted to give me a lot, I felt deep inside that I could not receive it.

Bert Hellinger describes this not being able to receive 'as the refusal of the depressed person to take, and that this can be traced back to a refusal to take from the father, the mother or both. This refusal is continued later on in relationships and manifests in having trouble receiving positive things. Some people say that they don't want to receive because what is offered to them is either not good enough or is not sufficient.
Others say that they cannot receive because something is wrong with the person who gives them something. Whatever the reason for the refusal is, the result is that someone will remain inactive and empty by not receiving anything.'*

The emptiness of the depression can often be casted back to a refusal to receive

---

To connect with someone else, it is necessary to be with yourself

Because I felt emotionally unsafe as a child - the invisible pain of my parents being constantly present - I unceasingly

---

* Bert Hellinger - *De wijsheid is voortdurend onderweg [Wisdom is Continuously On the Way]*

scanned the feelings of the people around me. In this way I became increasingly distant from my own feelings and from the experience of my body.

In the symbiotic relationship that I had with my mother, I was afraid that if I went too far away from her she would abandon me; not physically - she would never do that – but emotionally. If I were happy when she was not, I feared she would turn away from me emotionally. I therefore associated choosing my own path with being lonely .

When I learned in therapy groups that the only thing I had to do in contact with others was 'to be myself', this gave me a tremendous liberation and relief even though it was not easy and I had to learn it again.

The only thing I had to do in contact with others was 'to be myself'

When I started to focus on what I wanted myself, I didn't need to be continuously busy guarding my boundaries towards others; I automatically had enough space.

The nervous system comes into balance when we are connected to others

Just like plants that turn to the sunlight, every person needs the light of love and friendship. When this is lacking, we soon end up in fears and depressions.

Our society has become increasingly individualistic and we have partly lost the connection with Nature, our social network and our parents and ancestors. It is mainly due to the loss of these connections that rates of depression have become higher and higher.

In tests with rats it appears that the good or bad functioning of all important physiological systems of the body (heart rhythm, sleep, blood pressure, body temperature and the immune system) are related to the presence or absence of the loving presence of the mother. This also applies to humans.

When your parents responded with empathy to your emotional needs as a child, your ability to offer resistance against stress and depressions later in life is much stronger.

When your parents responded with empathy to your emotional needs as a child, your ability to offer resistance against stress and depressions later in life is much stronger

---

Psychiatrist Gradus van Florestein writes:

"When we know and feel ourselves connected to the larger whole, our depression ebbs away; we are in the big soul again then and we are back home: the home from which in fact we never left.

"What should the woman do without a husband, the man without a woman, the man without a friend, the woman without a girlfriend? What should the mother do without a child and the child without a mother? What should the father do without a child and the child without a father?

"Often we see depressions occur when the contact with the family of origin is broken, or when the father has left because he was no longer allowed by the mother to be a father any more. When the connection with our (fore-) parents has been broken, we lose strength and we are more vulnerable." *

It doesn't matter what is the focus of your love

When in gestalt therapy years ago I told my therapist that I didn't feel love for anything and anyone, she advised me to take care of something - a plant, for example, or an animal or a doll - because when you give energy and attention to something, a flow of love starts to rise.

When you give energy and attention to something, a flow of love starts to rise

---

At the time I resisted, and I ignored her advice. Years later I thought about it again and bought a cuddly animal; a grey mouse with small black beady eyes and dangling arms and legs. Magnets in the paws made sure that the mouse could cling to something. The mouse immediately started to be alive for me and because I didn't want to leave it alone when I was away from home, I also bought a small light brown monkey of the same size, who had magnets in his hands as well.

I took them with me when I went to India and they felt like real travelling companions. When I left my room I told them where I was going and when I came back I told them what I had experienced. And gradually there arose an ever stronger bond between me and the toy animals. When I was asleep they lay on my chest, their arms spread out wide on my body.

---

* Gradus van Florestein - *De Depressie vanuit Verschuivend Perspectief [Depression from a Shifting Perspective]*

Gradually my cuddly family expanded: a white rabbit and a rabbit with pink and white stripes, a big plush rabbit, a big black monkey, a white sheep, a small soft hedgehog, a bear, a pink elephant and a doll made by my niece. The more I told these animals each day what I was experiencing and the more hugs I gave them, the more they came to life and the firmer our connection became.

Today they are still there and I am always looking forward to going home and meeting them again.

There are people who can photograph auras (the energy fields surrounding a person), and an aura also appears to rise around an object you love (like a cuddly animal). Our love and attention affects not only people, but also animals, plants and objects.

Antoine de Saint-Exupéry describes this in the story of *The Little Prince*, who starts loving a rose:

"The little Prince lives on a small planet where he spends his time caring for the plants and flowers in his garden. 'It is a very monotonous work' he says, 'but very easy.' One day he sees a rose in his garden - a flower like he has never seen before. The prince falls in love with the mysterious rose, which he waters with devotion and shelters from the wind. But the flower is vain and wants more and more, and the prince becomes tired of her. He decides to leave the planet and to start discovering the universe.

"He is looking for knowledge and insight and sees all kinds of strange things on his travels. After visiting a few other planets he comes to the earth, where he finds a rose garden.

"Although the prince has left his rose, he still cares about her. Seeing the other roses makes him sad. He thought his rose was the only rose in the universe, but now he sees that there are hundreds.

"When he is near despair, he is called by a fox. The fox teaches the prince many wise lessons, but the most important one is about the rose that the prince has left behind. 'That rose is not just a rose' says the fox. 'She is very special because of everything you have given to her. It is the time you have devoted to the rose that makes her so special. You become forever responsible for what you grow. You are responsible for your rose.'

"When the prince is back in the rose garden, he thinks of the wisdom of the fox and says to the other roses: 'You are beautiful, but empty. Nobody would die for you. Of course, a casual passer-by may think that my rose just looks like you. But my rose is more important than all of you, because it is the rose that I watered, the rose that I put under glass and sheltered with a folding screen. Because she was the one for whom I killed caterpillars (except a few here and there for the butterflies). She was the one I listened to when she complained or bragged, or even when she said nothing at all. Because she is my rose.'"

It is the time you have devoted to the rose that makes it so special

---

I have heard Osho say that if you have difficulty in connecting, it is very hard to begin with people first. People are complex beings; every person has a complete history and all kinds of sensitivities. He says that you would be better to start building a relationship with a tree for example, or with an object. Neither a tree nor an object burdens you with their own history, yet an interaction with them can also start happening.

I love the story Osho once tells about a monk, who when travelling knocks at a temple door to ask for shelter for the night. The abbot opens the door and gives him permission to sleep in the temple. This temple is packed with hundreds of wooden Buddha statues. It is freezing cold and in the middle of the night the monk takes a Buddha statue and sets it on fire to warm himself up near the flames.

The next morning the abbot is very angry and asks the monk how he could do this: simply burn a Buddha. The monk says with astonishment that he didn't know that it was a Buddha and pokes with his staff in the ashes to find the bones. Furiously the abbot puts him out of the temple.

The following morning he sees the monk kneeling down in front of a concrete pole along the road. The monk has put flowers on and around the pole and honours it with great reverence. When the abbot asks what he is doing the monk says: "It doesn't matter what you worship; Buddha can be found in everything."

Buddha can be found in everything

In his book *Healing without Freud or Prozac* psychiatrist David Servan-Schreiber describes how he wrote the following advice in the medical records of a depressed elderly person who had undergone a bypass operation: "As far as the depression is concerned: the most beneficial for the patient would be to purchase a dog. If the patient claims that this is too much work, a cat is also possible, because it does not have to be walked. If that still seems too much to him, then a bird or a fish. And if the patient still refuses, a beautiful houseplant."

The medical world however was very dismissive of this and could not see that this was healing advice.

The psychiatrist tells of a study conducted in an old people's home which showed that the mortality rate dropped by half simply when the residents looked after a plant.

When I was depressed I noticed that there is an interaction between plants and human beings: all the plants in my apartment stopped flowering then, and their leaves hung limp and lifeless. They got bugs or other diseases. When I felt good again, the plants started to thrive and they bloomed out of season.

I am my own study object

When Meera Hashimoto invited me in the Art Therapist Training to see what it was I was doing in the way I contacted others and how I created my own isolation, I initially felt very alone. But at the same time I could feel her respect for me and her trust, because she was not going to help me by taking over the work I had to do. She believed in my capacity.

As I described already in the chapter 'the turning point in my depression', from that moment on I began to observe. I looked accurately at what I was doing in the contacts I had with the participants of the training. What I noticed was that I was too busy with myself. In fact, it was only 'I' 'I' 'I'; *I* am so sad, *I* feel so unhappy, *I* do not get what I want from life *I* don't know how to get out of my depression. I thought that everyone else felt only happy and sparkling. I was constantly angry at them and jealous, because I thought they knew how to live while I didn't. I used the people around me by expecting them to offer me a solution. And what they gave was never enough for me, so it was not surprising that they turned away from me.

I was angry at and jealous of other people

When I saw this, I started to behave differently. When someone gave me something -attention, a shared conversation, a smile, a hug - I really received it and was happy with it. Even when someone smiled and continued walking, I cherished the smile. When I caught myself thinking that, 'he is smiling though he doesn't mean it' I stopped that thought right away and stayed with the gratitude for the smile. Because I was receptive, the other person was also happy and it became an interaction. I started seeing more and more gifts every day.

I also started to ask about the other person out of interest. Previously I would simply act from an eagerness to please and the other person felt that immediately. Now I enquired into the other person from the realisation that he or she had exactly the same emotions as me, even if they weren't depressed (although I found out that many people laugh even when they are unhappy inside). I understood that the other also experienced all kind of things: anger, disappointment, hope, joy, desire, love, hate and despair. Our conversation was now on an equal level.

I started to feel that when I appreciated what I received and let go of the desire to get more, there was enough for me. I let go of the feeling that the other person had to give me what I had missed from my father and mother, and realised that no one could ever be my parent. But I could receive in small pieces from a lot of people what my parents had not been able to give me.

There was enough for me when I appreciated what I got

Only now that I realised I would never get from my parents what I had missed was I able to feel the pain of not having it. At the same time I was able to understand that they could not give certain things because of what they had experienced in their own lives.

Besides that I saw more and more how much they had given me and I was grateful.

The meditations that we did every day gave me a lot of insight and helped me to be able to stand alone in myself, so that I no longer had to cling to people for 'solutions'.

And then the miracle happened: people loved me and wanted to relate to me.

Contact Exercises

In the safety of the meditative and loving environment in Meera's training I dared to make real contact with myself and to face everything inside of me.

During the contact exercises we did, I felt that I could only connect with others when I was connected to myself.

I discovered that contact with people was simple when I was just myself.

Only when I was connected to myself
I could connect with others

One morning we did an exercise in which we had to dance in front of another person. I did my very best to make sure that my dance partner would enjoy dancing with me; I copied his movements and tried to answer his dance with my dance. My dance partner, however, moved further and further away from me.

Only later did I realise that as soon as I started to try to please the other person, I had lost contact with myself and so with them.

Later that morning, I was so happy with a beautiful painting that I had done that I danced out of pure joy. I didn't care what anyone would think of my dance. Spontaneously a woman danced with me and there was joy; our movements strengthened and enriched each other.

Looking at yourself

After this training I continue opening myself to others. I do not want to end up isolated anymore. Sometimes I still feel like an outsider. But the difference now is that I feel it very consciously and that I stay connected to myself in my feeling-excluded. I don't try to connect with somebody in a forced way, because this is the very point that would mean I were avoiding what is going on in me. In fact, usually I am not really excluded but something happens that triggers a painful experience from the past. By staying with it and consciously feeling the pain, the experience of the past starts healing. I don't bear a grudge for so long anymore after someone has hurt me.

Meera says in the Art Therapist Training:
"What you judge in the other, you are yourself. If you really understand this, you can forgive others and yourself.

The more you fight, the more you will be defeated. You end up in a suffering, which has no end. There is no end to darkness. We have to gather our consciousness. We cannot delay. If you delay, you create more fear, doubt, struggle, competition, jealousy. It is always you. So look at yourself in such a way; all arrows you put on others, put them back towards yourself. Outer conflict is inner conflict. If you always look at things like this and direct everything inside, you can see yourself clearly."

What is very important here is that you look at yourself with an attitude of love, compassion and understanding. If not, looking at yourself degenerates into self-rejection.

What you judge in the other you are yourself

Three ways of being in contact: the Camel, the Lion and the Child

We can be in contact with the other person in three ways: as the Camel, as the Lion or as the Child (where 'the Child' means being authentic, being in a space of meditation). Usually we have all three in us, but one of the three has the upper hand.

The Camel submits to the other and does what the other says. The Camel is a slave. That can be appealing because it is easy; you do not have to think about things yourself then. You feel you are pleasing the other with your docility, but in the end it starts to feel like a prison; you have no freedom.

The Lion revolts against this and starts rebelling against the other. He doesn't do what the other person says or even does just the opposite. That is a little more free-spirited than the Camel, but the Lion is still not free, because he is also bound in reaction to the other. His choices are not made of his own free will, but are only aimed at doing something that the other person doesn't want or which is contrary to the opinions of the other. He says 'no' because it gives him an identity.

The Child responds from within his or her own freedom. Even when instructed by the other person, the Child attends to his or her own inner feeling and impulse. The Child's behaviour may correspond with what the other person asks, be completely the opposite, or simply have nothing to do with it. The Child is the space of meditation. It is the most flexible position of the three. You are alone in this, completely dependent on yourself. You are not seeking any attention, either positive or negative, anymore.

In both the Camel and Lion positions you always depend on attention; you ensure that the other is there, either by following the other person (the Camel) or by fighting the other person (the Lion). We often don't follow our own energy because we want others to love us.

So the question is whether you are willing to be alone; whether you really do things from your centre; whether you follow what gives you joy in life.

This naturally raises fear and it is important not to suppress it. In the beginning it is very dark. In the beginning nobody comes to you. When you smile, no one comes. That is very dark. The only way is not to escape; to stay open and see where you are going as you find your original light. This is the work. You can remind yourself of this through meditation.

Only meditation can bring you into the space of the Child. You can't practise it. You can't act it. Only through meditation can you connect with what is inside, with what is good for you.

Meera indicates that 'trying' to make contact is the attitude of the Lion. Meera: 'Trying means that you resist the encounter deep inside. When you try something, in fact you don't *do* it. The Lion says: look, I'll do it, but I don't enjoy it. The Child never tries. If you are 'trying' to meet people they will run away from you because you are not authentic.'

"'What is REAL?' asked the Small Rabbit one day when they were lying next to each other, near the hearth in the nursery, before Nana came to tidy up. 'Does it mean that you have something inside that buzzes, and a catch from the outside?'

"'REAL is not how you are made,' said Leather Horse. 'It's something that happens to you. If a child loves you for a long, very long time, not just to play with you, but REALLY loves you, then you become REAL.'

"'Does that hurt?' asked the Rabbit.

"'Sometimes,' said the Leather Horse, because he always spoke the truth. 'If you are REAL, then you don't care that it has hurt.'

"'Does it all happen suddenly, just like being wound up?' he asked, 'or piece by piece?'

'It doesn't happen all at once,' said the Leather Horse. 'You just become it. It takes a long time. That's why it doesn't happen often with things that break easily, or have sharp edges, or should be treated very carefully. In general, by the time you become REAL, you are usually cuddled threadbare and your eyes have fallen out and your legs are dangling and you look ragged. But that doesn't matter, because once you are

REAL, you are not ugly anymore, except for people who don't understand it.'"*

If you are totally real, you are not ugly any more, except for people who don't understand it

---

The moment I feel *real* in connection with myself and the other, what I have been searching for all my life suddenly opens: my passion. The next chapter is about passion.

---

* Margery Williams - *Het Fluwelen Konijn [The Velveteen Rabbit]*

Part 7

Passion and Connection with the Soul

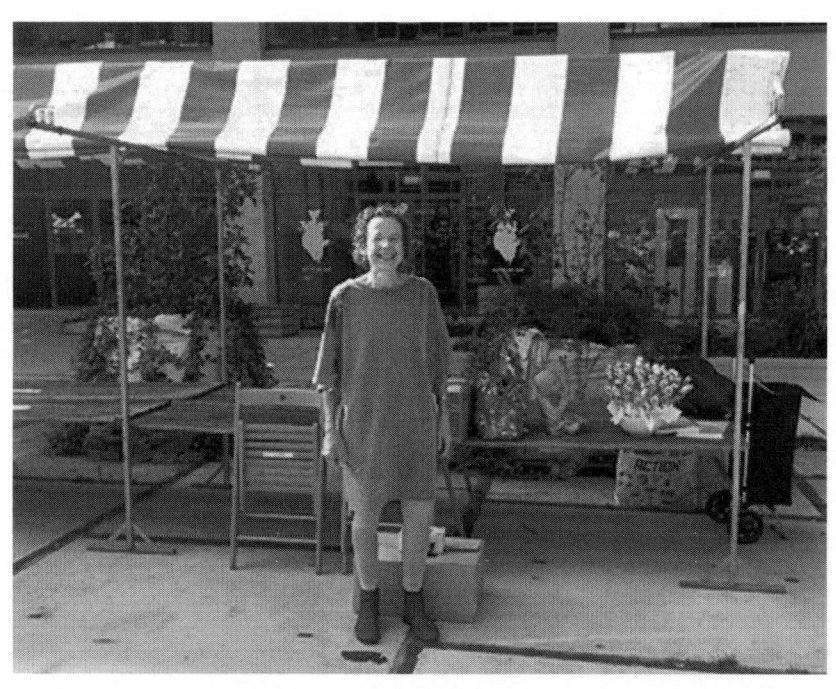

18 PASSION AND MEANING

The main reason for feelings of hopelessness and despair is not a lack of happiness, but a lack of meaning in life.

Emily Esfahani Smith

Your vocation is where your deepest joy and the need of the world meet.

Theologian Frederick Buechner

We are capable of unique things, all of us, but we need time to discover what they are. Our true potential is buried under so many layers. Only when the time is right we discover who we really should be or become.

Manjari Sharma, Artist

Since I was eleven I have been looking for my *vocation*. I heard my mother talk about her vocation: to become a primary school teacher. I imagine a vocation as a light that appears from above or as a voice that speaks to you from heaven. I watch and listen when I walk to school and return home at the end of the school day, but I don't hear or see anything.

I feel the strength that my mother's vocation has given her; a vision of the future that has caused her to survive the horrors of the concentration camp.

Even though I don't hear or see anything, I don't give up and keep on searching. Finally my vocation doesn't come in the form of a light or a voice, but as a feeling: it is the energy ball that jumps up in my upper stomach when the woman in Taizé tells me about the meditation centre of Osho in India. That feeling is the announcement of my passion - my vocation - and leads me to encounter the meaning of my life.

---

*The announcement of my passion
is a strong feeling in my upper stomach*

Meaning

Not being able to fulfil the need for meaning is a major cause of depression. I notice that throughout the whole history of my depression; as soon as I am busy with something that gives meaning to my life, my dejection disappears and when that meaningful activity ceases I become depressed again.

Emily Esfahani Smith writes in her book *De kracht van betekenis [The Power of Meaning]*, that experiencing meaning in life is more important than being happy. The Netherlands is called one of the happiest countries yet at the same time the depression rates are very high.

Emily explains that people describe themselves as happy if

they are not ill, have positive emotions and have enough money. The presence of all those things does not mean that they also experience meaning in their lives. It is very common that people, especially when they lack nothing in terms of physical health and material things, nevertheless experience their lives as meaningless. On the other hand, people who have none of this can experience their lives as meaningful when they are able to develop their talents, feel that they are meaningful to others and are involved with the people they live with.

Experiencing what you do as meaningful can mean you consider it worth the sacrifice to suspend your happiness for a period of time. Runners of a marathon endure pain and exhaustion to finish and parents deny themselves a lot for the happiness of their children (e.g. not going to the movies to help their child with homework). Meaning is perceived as more important than happiness.

I myself notice this when writing this book. For eight months I hardly leave my house, I work throughout the whole summer and I do not go out in the evening, to be fresh again the next morning for the writing process. But I have never liked waking up in the morning as much as I do in this period.

Meaning is perceived as more important than happiness

The Austrian psychiatrist Victor Frankl survived Nazi concentration camps. He tells in his book *Man's Search for Meaning* how - in order to survive in this desolate environment – he started looking for what could make his stay in these camps meaningful. His advice to people in desperate situations is not to ask life what it can do for you, but to always ask yourself what you can do for life. He found his freedom within the concentration camps by determining his own attitude to the difficult circumstances in which he found himself and by following his own path.

Don't ask in desperate situations what life can do for you, but always ask yourself what you can do for life

---

In her book *De kracht van betekenis [The Power of Meaning] Emily Esfahani Smith describes* how depression can disappear the moment you give meaning to the difficult situation in which you find yourself. Writing can be a good tool. The search for meaning alone is healing already. It turns out that even post-traumatic stress syndrome does not occur if people who have experienced a traumatic event can give meaning and significance to it.

For example, I have benefitted a lot when someone who gave a lecture about depression, called it 'a passage'. A passage to something new, even though you don't know yet what this 'new' is. The word 'passage' gave me the image of a dark tunnel with a light at the end. 'Passage' suddenly gave my depression a meaning: I was - even though it was unconscious - involved in the transition from one state of being to another.

When I told someone that, despite following so many therapy groups, I still ended up in my final depression, she said: 'You will have needed that depression to be able to write this book.' All of a sudden that last depression got so much more value.

Friedrich Nietzsche, a German poet and philosopher said: 'Whoever has a 'why' for which he can live, can tolerate almost every 'how''.

It does not matter in fact what kind of story you tell yourself to give meaning to your depression, so long as it's positive. When depressed, you tend to create a negative story about your life. This is often a pattern that has developed over the years. It has become a habit. You can reverse this; you can learn to tell a positive story about your life. It is not about repressing painful feelings. Even when you experience painful feelings, you can make a positive story out of it, for example by appreciating the fact that you are now beginning to feel the pain and that you are starting a process of healing.

You can learn to tell a positive story about your life

You yourself are what you have to give

Pamela Kribbe highlights in her book *Dark Night of the Soul* that you yourself are what you have to give. You yourself have done something with all that you have learnt and inside your being you've made something out of it that is yours; something which is unique to you.

When you give yourself, you're connected to everything around you and all at once things come to support you and give you the right circumstances to continue to express your energy in the world.

Pamela emphasizes the importance of the darkness in ourselves here:

"You give the highest of yourself the moment you are willing to connect with the lowest in yourself. With the lowest I mean: your fears, doubts, sombreness, in short the darkness that is in your soul as a result of unprocessed painful experiences.

The highest of yourself starts shining the moment you bend to the darkest part in yourself."*

* Pamela Kribbe - *Dark Night of the Soul*

*The highest of yourself starts shining
the moment you bend to the darkest part in yourself*

Exercises to get into the flow

I am convinced that you always come out of your depression the moment you find your passion and can go your unique way. To find it, you need to shake off what it has been covered by. For me, a lot of digging was needed for that.

It's no one's fault that so many conditionings from the past have buried us under everything that must and should be done. But there is a way through it, and when you get to your source, your fountain of life wells up with great force. Precisely because I have known the depression, I appreciate that fountain so much more.

The Osho® Born Again Meditation has been an important tool for me to get into the flow that has led me to my passion.
   I now describe three exercises that have also helped me to follow my life flow.

Creating a Collage

At the end of the schema therapy I am increasingly worried about the fact that I do not know yet what kind of work I will do next.
   My creative therapist suggests I find or draw for myself - without thinking of future work - pictures of what inspires

me, moves me, touches me, makes me happy or otherwise appeals to me, and make a collage of it.

That feels like a good idea, especially because I can completely suspend my thoughts about future work. I start right away. Browsing through a large stack of magazines, I immediately feel what attracts me or not, and so I begin to trust that I know what appeals to me. I group the images into different categories and use one large sheet per category.

On the first sheet I paste men, women and children who are doing something with every fibre of their being. Their eyes are shining. You can see that they have lost all sense of time in what they do.

The second sheet is filled with images of people meditating in beautiful places in Nature; people sitting in lotus position on rocks that protrude above the sea, and monks in orange robes, walking serenely behind each other. The sheet radiates a determination to reach the inner space - in a beautiful environment, with like-minded people.

On the third sheet there is a large white desk with an alarm clock on it: this desk radiates action and a desire to work. On that sheet I also paste a picture of a gate that is invitingly open to receive people.

On a fourth sheet I make drawings myself, of people who meditate in all kinds of situations: in an open train, listening to the sounds around them and enjoying the sun - sitting on a rock - and dancing and singing in the night with moon and stars.

While working on these sheets my energy starts to flow. It gives me a warm and happy feeling. When I look at my collage, I see that on the inside I know very well what I want: to share Active Meditations with dance, song and silence, in which all the senses are activated: better hearing, sharper vision, more feeling, more enjoyment and at the same time, becoming more and more quiet inside.

When I look at my collage, I notice that on the inside I know very well what I want

One thing is missing and that is the accomplishment of what I want.

Patrick Roozemond writes in his eBook *Start vanuit je Hart [Start from your Heart]:* "You cannot cultivate courage. You just need to look honestly at your inner saboteur who keeps you from taking a step. That is courage. Courage is to face your fears honestly and take action from there. You see your saboteur with the underlying fear and you take a step. Acknowledged fear becomes courage." *

Courage is facing your fears honestly and taking action from there

---

* Patrick Roozemond - *Start vanuit je Hart [Start from your Heart]*

Doing Something New

One day during my depression I break through the routine of 'doing the same thing every day' by buying a new salt and pepper set in a small shop; two funny characters, which I put on show in my kitchen. Suddenly my whole house has a different look; my apartment is no longer the same and contains something that is really mine, something that is connected to my taste. This is such a good feeling that I am prompted to do something else that's new for me. I remember the delicious smell of fresh bread that tickled my nose when I cycled home. Decisively I go to the bakery and find a kind of hot roll which I have never tried before and enjoy the new taste. This is a day that has made me really happy.

During my depression I always thought that something big had to happen to get me out of it. Now I start to feel that happiness is in small things and that new things bring me to life.

I start to feel that happiness is in small things and that new things bring me to life

---

Making a Mandala

For me, making a mandala is at the same time both a relaxed and a powerful way to follow myself from within. It is also healing; both in creating it and in looking at it. If I am dealing with difficult things or strong emotions, working on a mandala calms me down.

These effects only happen when I design the mandala myself and not if I colour-in a pre-drawn mandala.

Making the mandala goes like this:

You need a blank sheet of paper and a set of coloured pencils. It is more pleasing if you have coloured pencils with beautiful, deep colours. I'm a fan of the Staedtler brand. Then you choose the colour which most attracts you right then and draw something in the middle of the sheet: a circle, a flower, a square, a triangle; it can be anything. Then you take another colour that appeals to you and connect a new figure to the one you have already drawn in the middle. You repeat this new figure around the central one in as many directions as you like. Then you take the next colour that appeals to you and continue to attach something new to the already existing pattern, which you repeat in the same number of directions.

You are not going to judge what you have made; if you have judgements, you let go of them.

Sometimes my mandala consists of bright, cheerful colours and I suddenly feel like using black or gray. My mind then says, "What a waste of my beautiful mandala, now it will become very dull." Yet I follow my original feeling and continue with black or grey; I want to stay true to following my impulses. And the crazy thing is that whatever comes into being is always beautiful. That makes me trust more and more that everything belongs to life and that the whole is precious.

Mistakes are also part of the mandala; you leave these uncorrected - you do not eliminate them. This also works in my life: when I simply accept my mistakes and even see the beauty of them, I am much more free.

> *When I simply also accept my mistakes,*
> *I am much more free*

Making the mandala helps me to follow my impulses; to trust in something that does not come from my mind. While drawing and colouring, I see that something beautiful is unfolding without me having that intention. For me it also helps me sleep when I do it before going to bed.

You can also embroider the mandala, in which case a lot more patience is needed, or you can create one in the forest with pine cones and twigs, leaves and stones - or with seashells on the beach.

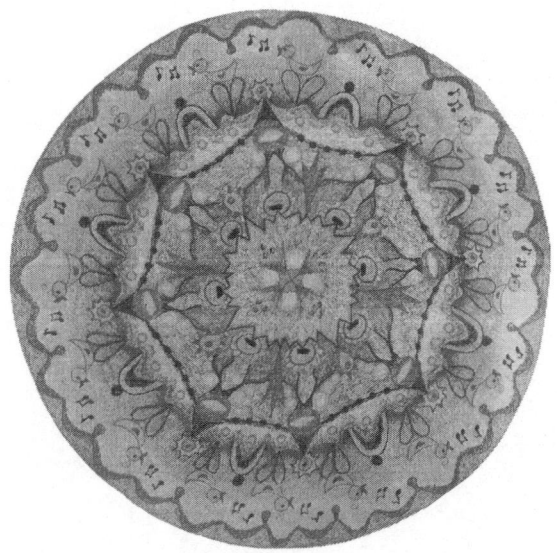

All these exercises have helped me to follow what is already present deep inside. The more I follow myself, the more I understand the voice of my soul.

Depression is a message, an invitation from the soul. This is the subject of the next chapter.

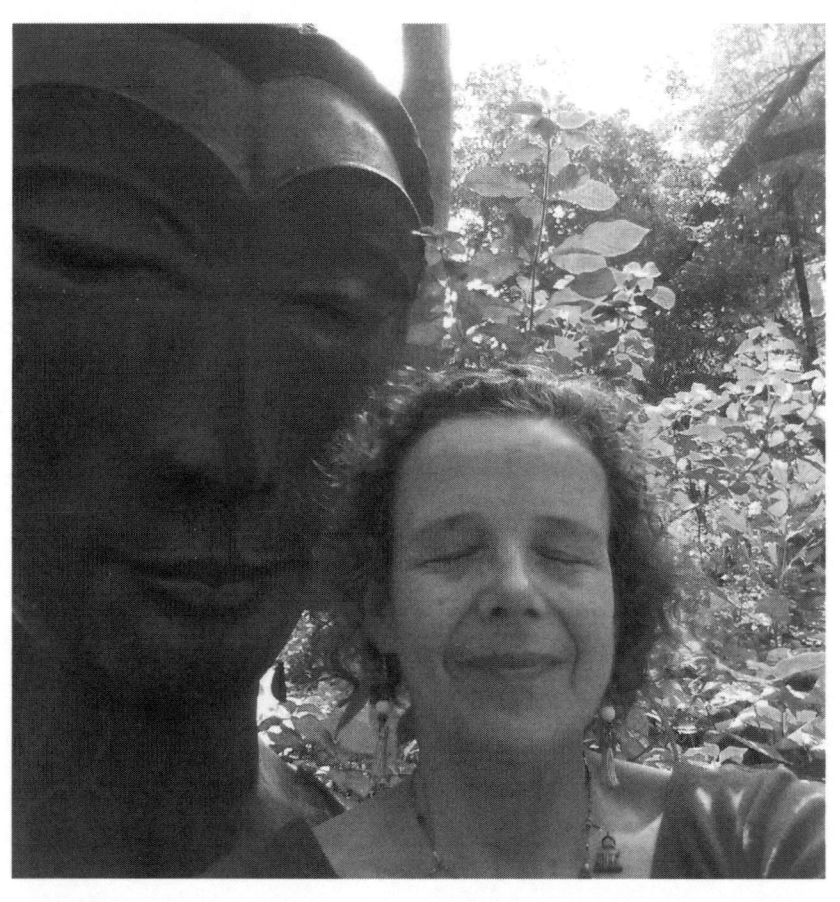

19 LISTENING TO YOUR SOUL

Almost everyone has resistance against experiences of great loss or pain. You can then often only be reborn through a Night of the Soul and start experiencing life in a new and different way. During the Night your fear, your mistrust or your bitterness are fully magnified. This gives you the chance to fully understand these moods and sink into them so deeply that at a given moment you decide that it is unbearable and it has to be different. Eventually you get out of it. Eventually the opposing part in you bows to something bigger than itself. It starts opening to love.*

Pamela Kribbe

Depression: a message from the Soul

Psychiatry often does not assume that depression has something to tell us, that it is based on a message: the message from our soul.

The soul invites us to see the shadow sides that we have repressed most deeply and to integrate them into our lives so that we can be complete and don't have to suppress anything anymore.

---

* Pamela Kribbe - *Dark Night of the Soul*

> *Depression is founded on a message from our Soul*

Pamela Kribbe describes in her book *Dark Night of the Soul* the deeper meaning of depression from the perspective of the soul:

"During this life and the many lives before, you have experienced a lot of pain and disappointment, which at the soul level may have created a deep 'no' to life. Often you are not aware of that. You have tried in many ways (in your work, in your family life, with friends) to find distractions from this 'no' and from the deep despair and hopelessness that go along with it. But the soul asks to face these deeply hidden feelings. To look at them and to feel them in the roots. Only then a transformation can happen and the negative feelings can be turned into light and life force.

In America 'hit rock bottom' is a well-known expression. Go to the ground, to the bottom of the abyss, for only then can you drop off from there to life and positivity."

> *Only if you can face deeply hidden feelings transformation can happen*

In one of his performances, Stef Bos tells us that he lived near a huge river with large whirlpools. His mother always told him: 'If you ever end up in a vortex, let yourself go with it all the way to the bottom of the river and then move off.' This is a metaphor for depression: when you no longer resist it, space is created for you to take a new direction.

It is almost impossible for me to make a connection with my soul when I am depressed. Gradus van Florestein - a psychiatrist who pays attention to the soul during his treatments – sees this in the depressed people he guides too: 'When we are gloomy or depressed, we have also lost a part of our soul. In severe cases we have to a large degree lost the very connection with our soul. When we are either insufficiently or not at all on the path of our soul, we become unhappy and depressed.'*

> *When we are either insufficiently or not at all on the path of our soul, we become unhappy and depressed*

The Path of the Soul

Pamela Kribbe describes the darkness one is going through in depression as a way of transforming oneself; how one wants to go deep inside to let go of the old and to be able to be born again.

I quote:

"I consider the Night of the Soul as a journey of transformation of consciousness, in which the unknown and the darkness come to the fore and the known is left behind. This journey leads to a new birth, but not without birth contractions that touch you to your very core and force you to let go of old certainties.

"On the path of the soul you are basically attracting difficult situations and difficult relationships with people from an inner level, because deep down you want to come to a deeper self-understanding. This way you can face deep fears and false images and you can go beyond them.

---

* Gradus van Florestein - *De Depressie vanuit Verschuivend Perspectief [Depression from a Shifting Perspective]*

The night of the soul is a transformation of consciousness

"Although it appears in the depression that your soul is unreachable, yet it never leaves you. The moment you dare to receive the darkness inside yourself, you will start to feel the connection with your soul again.

"By your environment you are often exhorted to be strong, to put yourself together and continue in the old way. Thereby you are encouraged to move away from your dark feelings, whereas it is in fact necessary to face them and not to be alienated from a part of yourself that is also yours.

"Realise that you ignite the greatest light within yourself if you are willing to bow to the darkest, most neglected parts inside yourself."*

Reincarnation

Until I was thirty, I was not concerned with the concept of reincarnation. I came across it for the first time during my gestalt therapy training. When I returned from the toilet on one of the training days, the conversation happened to be about this subject. My teacher asked me, 'Who were you in your past life?' When I looked at her with wide eyes - I had never assumed a past life - she asked me smilingly: 'Or are you completely new here?' 'No,' I said immediately, to my own surprise. From that moment on I opened myself to the possibility of past lives, and a little later I got short glimpses of them for the first time. The feeling that I had was that of a sort of 'knowing'.

---

* Pamela Kribbe - *Dark Night of the Soul*

A year later I did a breath training at the Osho International Meditation Resort in India, during which - in an exercise – I made contact with the moment of my incarnation in this life. I felt that before my birth I was in a peaceful, wide space in the universe when my mother suddenly called me to come to Earth. I did not feel ready for it yet. Her call was so strong, however, that I gave in and moved to her womb while retaining a sense of 'no' at the same time. That 'no' came from things from past lives - although I do not know what those things are - and caused me not to dare surrender to another life on Earth, with all the pain and complications that come with it. Notwithstanding this, my 'yes' was bigger, otherwise I would not have come.

I did not feel ready yet to come to Earth

Now I can see that I had unconsciously to apply the brakes to myself because the unwillingness to live which I had brought with me at birth wanted to be heard and seen, and my depressions were the vehicle for that.

The depressions have shown me how much darkness, negativity, fear, despair, disappointment and hopelessness were present in me. Finally I had to give up my ego - which wanted to stand above everything. That has become my salvation and has caused my movement towards the light.

Depression, a Steppingstone towards Bliss

By reaching the very bottom in my last depression, I was able to move myself upwards to the light and from that moment my consciousness has permanently changed. Now I am grateful, go along with the flow of life, follow my passion, have an understanding for others and for myself, feel more humble and am connected to the Earth for the first time, enjoying everything that can be felt and experienced on this planet, with a deep respect for life and connected with life after death. Now I feel joy and satisfaction every day and simple actions are filled with meaning. I love life. My depression has been a stepping-stone towards bliss.

Every day I use the useful tools which I have collected in therapies, trainings and especially through my life experience and which I have described in this book. I use them to meet the challenges of daily life. Although they are not always easy, I am finally grateful for these challenges, because they make my growth possible.

Love

The most essential thing that has changed in me is that now I love myself.

Osho:
"Buddha says, *Love yourself...* This can become the foundation of a radical transformation. Don't be afraid of loving yourself. Love totally, and you will be surprised: The day you can get rid of all self-condemnation, self-disrespect - the day you can get rid of the idea of original sin, the day you can think of yourself as worthy and loved by existence - will be a day of great blessing. From that day onward you will start seeing people in their true light, and you will have compassion. And it will not be a cultivated compassion; it will be a natural, spontaneous flow.

"And a person who loves himself can easily become meditative, because meditation means being with yourself. If you hate yourself - as you do, as you have been told to do and you have been following it religiously - if you hate yourself, how can you be with yourself? And meditation is nothing but enjoying your beautiful aloneness. Celebrating yourself; that's what meditation is all about.

"Meditation is not a relationship; the other is not needed at all, one is enough unto oneself. One is bathed in one's own glory, bathed in one's own light. One is simply joyous because one is alive, because one is."*

---

* Osho - *Love, Freedom and Aloneness #2*

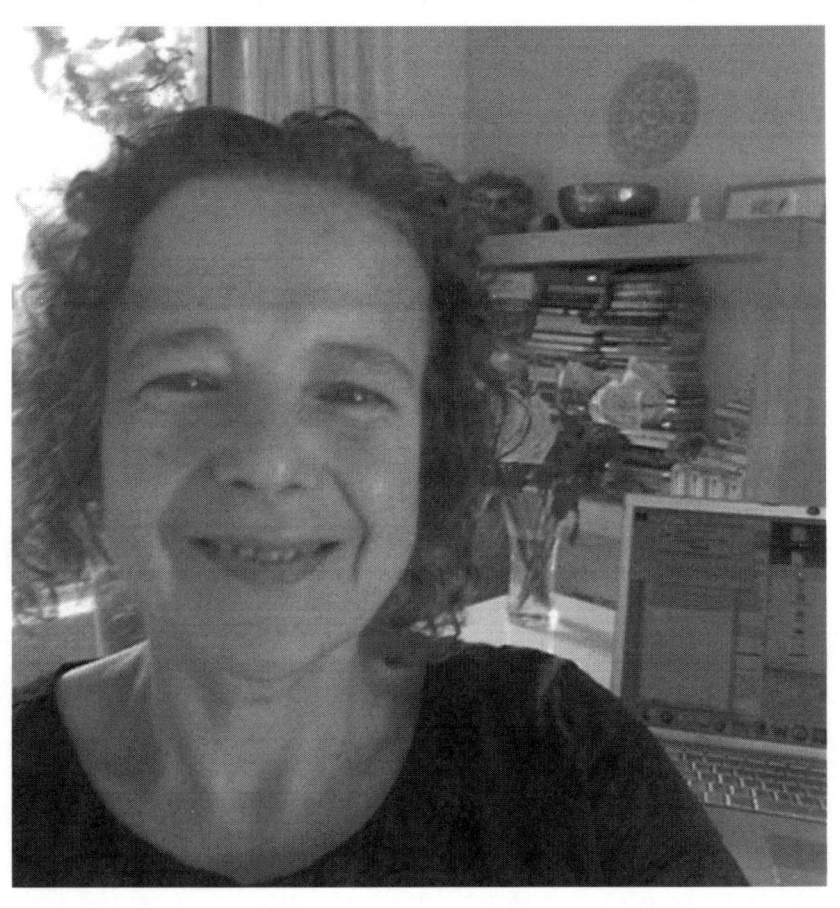

LAST WORD

When I was depressed I looked everywhere to find a book which spoke about how to come out of depression with consciousness; a book in which meditation would be an important part. I have now written the book I was looking for.

I know how difficult it is to get moving from the frozen state of depression. And I know how important it is to be recognised and accepted in the darkness in which you find yourself. That darkness has value, however, because it forms the foundation from which the light can arise.

How to continue?

The guidelines described in the various chapters can all lead you to initiate the flow of your own life.

It may be that one chapter appeals to you and another not at all.

My invitation is that when something from this book appeals to you, you build that into your day and make it a commitment to yourself.

Depression has often been a months-long or year-long exercise in negative thinking, in physically moving very little, in having not much contact with yourself or with others and of denying your body. This means that there is also a need for months or years of exercise to establish a life-affirming path again. I myself have experienced that when I said, 'yes' to this, practising it became so precious to me that I do not want to stop it any more - even now that I feel happy again.

It has been very supportive for me to write daily everything in a diary before going to bed. This prevents you from giving too much weight to one thing from the day. The way you write is important, too. It's very usual when you're depressed to tell your life story in a negative way, but when you start to write in a way that gives meaning to what you have experienced, a stream of 'giving meaning to your life' is put in motion. Even feeling pain can be meaningful when you describe it in terms like: 'I have the courage to feel the pain now, which allows it to heal.'

If you want to get started with the guidelines from this book, you may also encounter scepticism in yourself or in people around you.

The mind is always full of judgements and is often afraid of change or of opening up to something new. We have the choice to either listen to the mind or to take on the challenge of experimenting with new things. I have noticed that even a negative experience is better than maintaining the routine of 'the same every day'.

Maybe you dare not give up the antidepressants yet, do not believe in reincarnation, are afraid that meditation is vague, do not want to give up coffee with a lot of sugar, find family constellations a bit odd and hate connecting with others because you feel that everyone lets you down.

Nonetheless, there is something in you that has picked up this book. That might be the hand of your heart, of your inner child or of your soul. I think that many people who are depressed follow the invitation of their soul to stop everything in their lives for a while, to find that which is pure and true.

Each chapter contains a key that fits a door that can form an entrance to blissfulness. When you go through that door, it's possible you could first encounter a lot of pain; pain that still wants to be felt. If you dare to face it and then do not give up, that same pain will purify you. I say this from my own experience.

Never think that blissfulness is not for you; it is your birthright.
    At the most, the layers that cover blissfulness are somewhat thicker in one person than in another. But the thicker the layer you are going through, the greater the blissfulness that awaits you.

I wish you a good journey to your own life source.

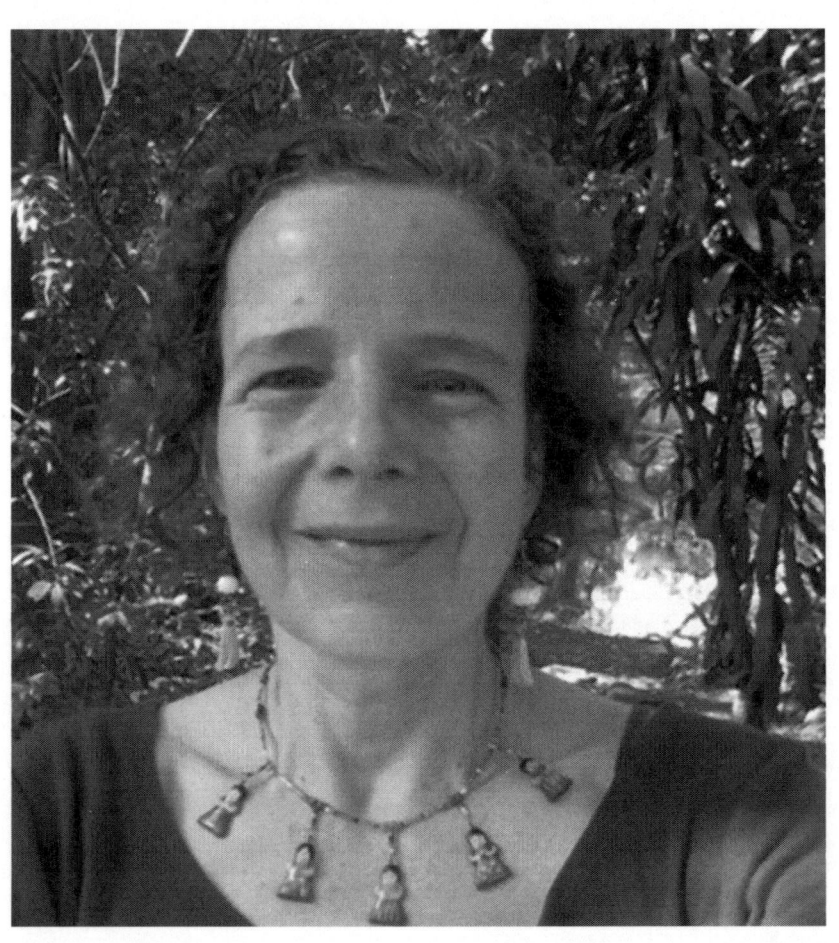

ABOUT THE AUTHOR

I, Modita (1962) have not practiced as a medical doctor since 2013, in order to fully devote myself to sharing the Active Meditations and Meditative Therapies of the Indian mystic Osho. I give individual consultations and an online course 'Beyond Depression with Consciousness'. I also facilitate Family Constellations and give the rejuvenating and deeply relaxing Japanese Therapeutic Face Massage.

My gratitude in overcoming my depression definitively is the main motivation I have for wanting to be a travel companion to everyone who wants to come out of his or her depression through consciousness.

See for more information:

- www.genietenvanmeditatie.nl [enjoyingmeditation] (the website is translated in English)
- www.voorbijdepressiemetmeditatie.nl [beyonddepression-withmeditation] (the website is translated in English)
- YouTube: Actieve Osho Meditaties
- Facebook: JoyinMeditation
- LinkedIn: Modita Van Zummeren

Email: info@genietenvanmeditatie.nl

If you want to receive my monthly newsletter, please send me an e-mail.

By invitation I give interactive lectures about how depression can become a stepping-stone towards bliss.

If you have questions or comments about this book or would like to share something personal, you can mail me.

WORD OF THANKS

Many beautiful people have contributed to this book, who I would like to thank here.

First of all I want to thank my parents for giving me life and for welcoming me into this world. I thank them for their love, strength, integrity, courage, wisdom, perseverance and the unremitting care they have had for me.

I thank Osho, my beloved master, for his invitation to my deepest core to live my truth and to be myself. For his wisdom, his humour and the many inner operations he has carried out with me. For touching the truth which was already present deep inside of me, but which was covered by many layers of dust. And for the inspiration he gives me every day.

I thank Meera Hashimoto for arousing my creativity and courage to do new things. For her invitation to connect with others and to learn from the other. For her sincere connection with Osho and for the transfer of his work. She is and will always be a source of inspiration for my work. I thank her for her contribution to overcoming my last depression. One month before she left the body I told her that I would mention her in my book and she smiled.

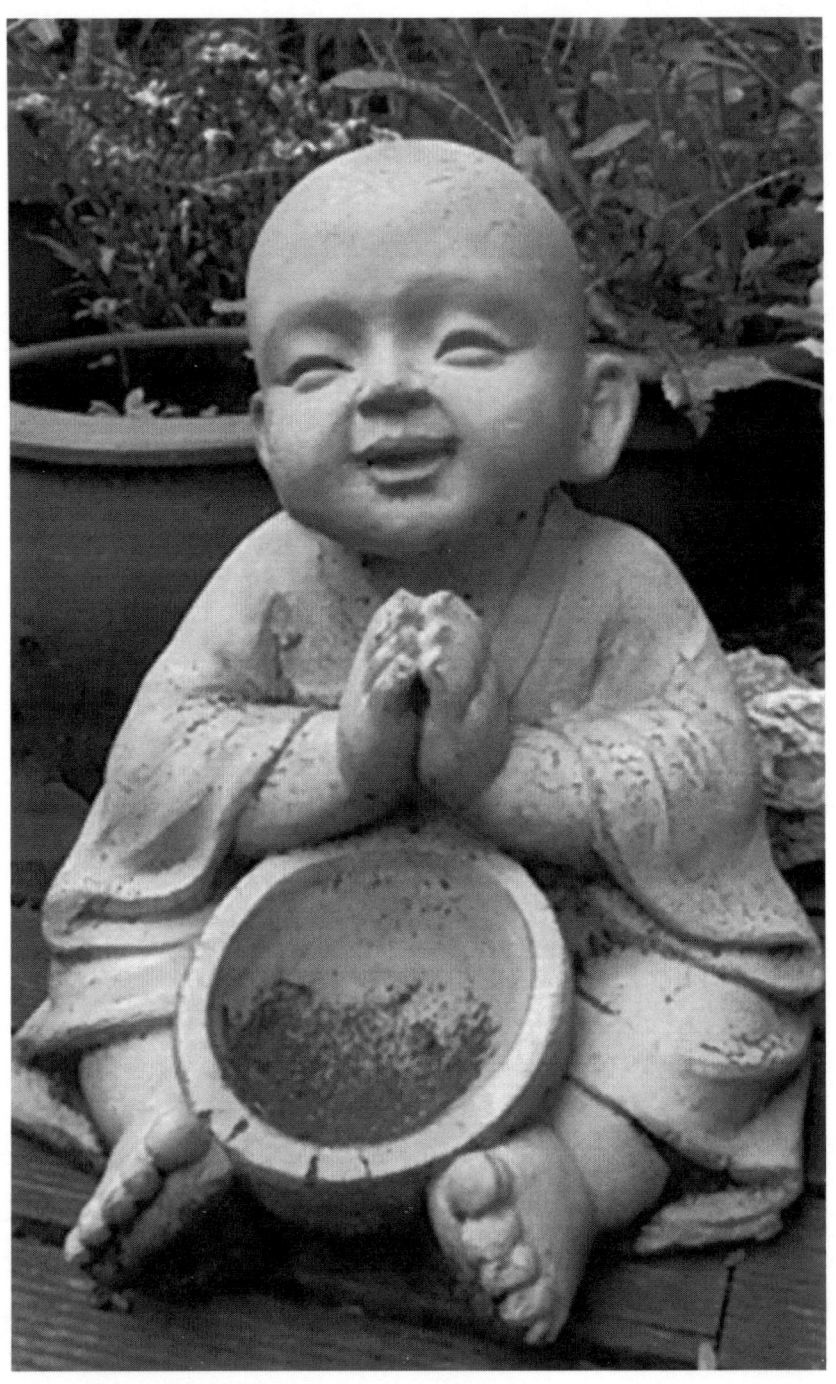

I thank my beloved friend Paripurna. For his friendship, his abundance, the devotion to the work he does in the Osho International Meditation Resort in Pune, for the devotion in his meditations, his honesty and humour. For his contribution to my growth, through everything that we have encountered in our relationship. And for the inspiration he is for my work.

I thank my sisters Lisette, Ingrid and Margo for always believing in me, no matter what happens. For growing with me. For the fact that they have always accepted me during my depressions and have continued to support me. And for sharing their joy of life with me.

I thank my unborn twin sister for the help she has given me to come to this Earth, for the intimacy that we have had together in the womb and for her presence in my life.

I thank the people of publishing company Aspekt for the careful and enthusiastic way in which they have published my book. I am particularly grateful to Mr Pierik Senior for the amiable and encouraging words he has given me during the entire process of editing, to Mark Heuveling for his patience, creativity and dedication with the design and layout of this book and to Sylvia Kamerbeek for her good organization.

I thank Bodhigita Jane Marshall for the beautiful corrections - with so much care and dedication - which turned my translation into fluent English.

I thank those who have contributed to a greater depth of this Book: Osho, Meera Hashimoto, Svagito Liebermeister, Bert Hellinger, Gradus van Florestein, Pamela Kribbe, Marjolein

Dubbers, Fons Delnooz, Patricia Martinot, Willem van de Sanden, David Servan-Schreiber, Peter Gøtzsche and Emily Esfahani Smith.

I thank Imke Bartels for her encouraging, enthusiastic support.

I thank Elena Donskaia for the inspiration she has given me during our many conversations, for her trust in my book and for her support.

I thank my aunt Marietje, for her unconditional trust in me and in my parents.

I thank Adriana van Roosmale, my dear friend, with whom I can share everything and who gives me so much inspiration.

I thank Frans Muskens, who has coached me in such a great way in giving shape to my company 'Joy in Meditation' and who initiated the spark in me for writing this book.

I thank Svagito Liebermeister, husband of Meera Hashimoto, who has given me so much depth with the training Family Constellation.

I thank Anja Rombouts, therapist at the mental health care in Eindhoven, for her belief in me, for bringing me back again and again to my *being* and for her continuously referring to the light in myself.

I thank therapists Ed Thelosen, Natasha, Brigitte, Theo and Diana of the mental health care in Eindhoven for everything they have given me, with so much patience and dedication, in the schema therapy. I thank them for their trust in my strength.

I thank my group members of the schema therapy: Lia, Orsha, Tanja, Ankie, Mirjam, Susan, Brigitte, Rudi, Marjanne and Ilse. For their trust in me, their support, humour and valuable feedback.

I thank Anita Joling for the guidance she has given me to find a way to share the meditations of Osho.

I thank Garimo Ackermann and Pramod Steeg for their care in reviewing the chapters on Osho meditations, so that the original words of Osho in the description of the meditations are guaranteed.

I thank Lisette Thooft for her feedback on the first pages of my book.

I thank Tosho, my Japanese friend, for his support throughout my depressions, for the energetic work he has done with me at a distance, for his love and his never ending trust in me.

And I thank myself, for never having given up and for always having continued searching to find my source.

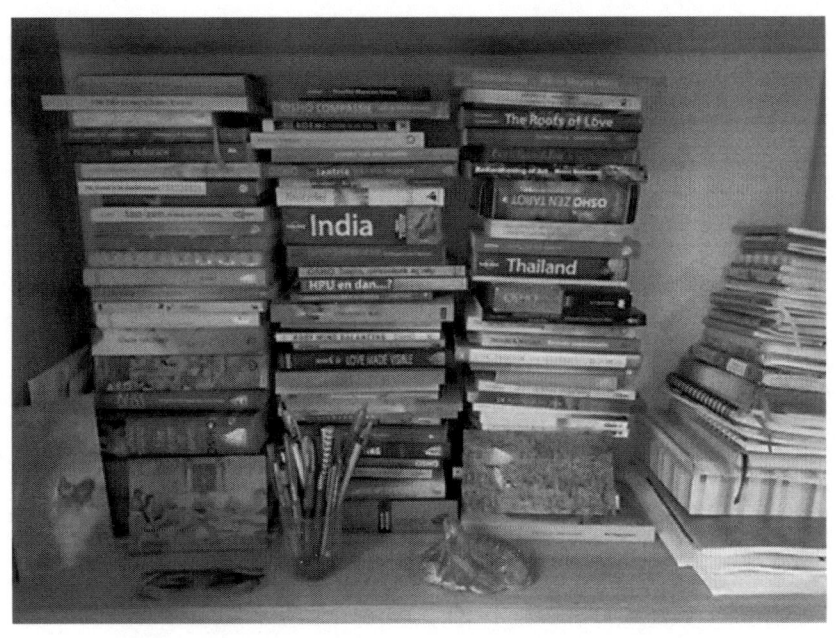

SELECTED BIBLIOGRAPHY

Book and Documentary about the dangers of Antidepressants:
* *Deadly Psychiatry and Organised Denial*, Peter C. Gøtzsche, Peter C. Gøtzsche og People's Press, Copenhagen 2015
* *'The Secrets of Seroxat'*, Panorama Documentary (BBC 2012)

Book about Anorexia Nervosa:
* *The Golden Cage*, Hilde Bruch, Harvard University Press, 1978

Book about moving towards the Light:
* *Spirituele Verdieping [Spiritual Deepening]*, Fons Delnooz & Patricia Martinot, Ankh-Hermes, 2003

Books by Osho:
* *Absolute Tao*, Osho, Osho International Foundation
* *Ancient Music in the Pines*, Osho, Osho International Foundation
* *The Art of Dying*, Osho, Osho International Foundation
* *Beloved of my Heart*, Osho, Osho International Foundation
* *Body/Mind Balancing*, Osho, Osho Publicaties, 2004
* *The Book of Wisdom*, Osho. Osho International Foundation

- *The Buddha; the Emptiness of the Heart*, Osho, Osho International Foundation
- *Come Follow To You*, Osho, Osho International Foundation
- *The Dhammapada: The Way of the Buddha*, Osho, Osho International Foundation
- *The Discipline of Transcendence*, Osho, Osho International Foundation
- *Don't Bite my Finger, Look where I am Pointing*, Osho, Osho International Foundation
- *The Fish in the Sea is Not Thirsty*, Osho, Osho International Foundation
- *From Darkness to Light*, Osho, Osho International Foundation
- *The Great Pilgrimage: From Here to Here*, Osho, Osho World Galleria
- *The Hidden Splendor*, Osho, Osho International Foundation
- *Intimacy, Trusting Oneself and the Other*, Osho, Osho International Foundation
- *Love, Freedom and Aloneness*, Osho, Osho International Foundation
- *The Message Beyond Words*, Osho, Osho International Foundation
- *My Way, The Way of the White Clouds*, Osho, Osho International Foundation
- *The New Alchemy: To Turn You On #8*, Osho, Osho International Foundation
- *The New Dawn*, Osho, Osho International Foundation
- *Om Mani Padme Hum*, Osho, Osho International Foundation
- *Osho Meditatie Handboek, Vrij zijn in het Hier & Nu [Osho Meditation Handbook. Being Free in the Here &*

Now], Osho, Osho Publikaties Nederland 2002
* *Beyond Psychology*, Osho, Osho International Foundation
* *The Path of the Mystic*, Osho, Osho International Foundation
* *The Rebellious Spirit*, Osho, Osho International Foundation
* *Sat Chit Anand,* Osho, Osho International Foundation
* *Satyam Shivam Sundram*, Osho, Osho International Foundation
* *The Supreme Doctrine,* Osho, Osho International Foundation
* *A Sudden Clash of Thunder,* Osho, Osho International Foundation
* *Tao: The Three Treasures*, Osho, Osho International Foundation
* *This Is It*, Osho, Osho International Foundation
* *Yoga: A New Directioin (Yoga: The Alpha and the Omega Vol 5) #2*, Osho, Osho International Foundation

Website Osho Meditation Center Pune:
* Osho International Meditation Resort www.osho.com
* Audio and video instructions for the OSHO Active Meditations: www.osho.com and www.imeditate.osho.com

Book about Osho Art Therapy from Meera Hashimoto:
* *ReAwakening of Art*, Meera Hashimoto, Perfect Publishers Ltd, 2005

Books about Family Constellations:
* *The Roots of Love*, Svagito Liebermeister, Perfect Publishers Ltd, 2006
* *Acknowledging What Is, Bert Hellinger in Conversation with Gabriele ten Hövel*, Publisher Het Noorderlicht, 2015
* *De wijsheid is voortdurend onderweg [Wisdom is Continuously on the Way]*, Bert Hellinger, Het Noorderlicht, 2012

Books and websites about Nourishment:
* *Voeding en Spiritualiteit [Food and Spirituality]*, Fons Delnooz & Patricia Martinot, Ankh-Hermes, 2002
* *Het Energieke Vrouwen Voedingskompas [The Energetic Women's Nutritional Compass]*, Marjolein Dubbers, Kosmos Uitgevers, 2016 and website: energiekevrouwenacademie.nl (in Dutch)
* *Food Pharmacy*, Lina Nerthby Aurell & Mia Clase, Bonnier Fakta, 2017
* Website Dr Mercola: www.mercola.com
* Website 'Arts en Voeding' [Doctor and Nourishment]: www.voedingonline.nl (in Dutch)

Book about vanishing twin syndrome:
* *The Surviving Twin Syndrome - Drama in the Womb*, Alfred Austermann & Bettina Austermann, 2008. Information: ifosys@msn.com

Workbook to overcome Depression
* *Depressie actief overwinnen [Active Overcoming Depression]*, Willem van de Sanden, Pearson, 1995

Books about Depression and Mourning:
* *Dark Night of the Soul*, Pamela Kribbe, www.amazon.co.uk, 2013
* *De Depressie Vanuit Verschuivend Perspectief [The Depression from a Shifting Perspective]*, Gradus van Florestein, Uitgeverij Akasha, 2009

* *Healing without Freud or Prozac*, Dr David Servan-Schreiber, Rodale International, 2004
* *Pil [Pill]*, Mike Boddé, Nijgh & van Ditmar, 2010
* *The New Black, Mourning, Melancholia and Depression*, Darian Leader, Penguin Books Ltd 2008

Book about Inner Child Work:
* *Je eigen-wijze weg [Your Self-Willed Way]*, Omkar Dingjan & Divyam Kranenburg, Aumm, 2012

Books about finding Meaning in your life:
* *De kracht van betekenis [the Power of Meaning]*, Emily Esfahani Smith, Uitgeverij ten Have, 2017
* *Man's Search for Meaning*, Viktor E. Frankl, Houghton Mifflin, 2006

Book about High Sensitivity
* *Handbook of Energetic Protection*, Fons Delnooz and Patricia Martinot, Independently published, 2015

E-book for free about starting a Company from your Idea:
* *Start vanuit je Hart [Start from your Heart]*, Patrick Roozemond, Stichting Pulsar Fonds, 2007

Trailer for documentary film about second generation war victims:
* Trailer *Buitenkampers, Boekan Main, Boekan Main! [People who lived outside the Japanese concentration camps, Boekan Main, Boekan Main!]* by Hetty Naaijkens- Retel Helmrich. www.buitenkampers.nl/portal/site/buitenkampers